ELECTROCARDIOGRAPHY FOR THE ANAESTHETIST

ELECTROCARDIOGRAPHY FOR THE ANAESTHETIST

W. N. ROLLASON

M.B. M.R.C.S. D.A. F.F.A.R.C.S.

Head of Department of Anaesthetics
The Royal Infirmary and University of Aberdeen

WITH A FOREWORD BY

WILLIAM W. MUSHIN

M.A., M.B. B.S. F.F.A.R.C.S.
(HON.)F.F.A.R.A.C.S. F.F.A.R.C.S.I. F.F.A.(S.A.)

Professor of Anaesthetics
Welsh National School of Medicine

SECOND EDITION

BLACKWELL SCIENTIFIC PUBLICATIONS
OXFORD AND EDINBURGH

©BLACKWELL SCIENTIFIC PUBLICATIONS 1964, 1969

*This book is copyright. It may not be reproduced by any means
in whole or in part without permission. Application with
regard to copyright should be addressed to the publishers.*

SBN 632 03510 2

FIRST PUBLISHED 1964

SECOND EDITION 1969

Printed in Great Britain by
ADLARD & SON LTD, THE BARTHOLOMEW PRESS, DORKING
and bound by
THE KEMP HALL BINDERY, OXFORD

TO MY WIFE

The good provider of that inestimable thing
a happy and a tranquil home

CONTENTS

FOREWORD

If the anaesthetist is to take notice of physiological changes in his patient and to relate his activities to them in a reasonable and flexible manner, he must receive continuous, reliable and quantitative information about these changes. The scientific instrument industry has been sensitive to this need and has responded quickly. There are now available highly developed devices for monitoring the main physiological systems of the body.

The problem facing the anaesthetist is interpretation. The barriers which have grown up round each field of medical knowledge often effectively prevent even basic information and terminology flowing readily from one field to another. It is essential and pressing that these barriers be broken down if the full benefit of the great advances in medical science be available to all who need them.

Electrocardiography is an example of this problem. The display and the recording of the electrical changes within the heart and their interpretation in terms of function and disease, is now widely practised and elaborate instruments to this end are readily available. Interested physicians all over the world devote their lives to a study of this matter and have developed great expertise and interpretive skill. The anaesthetist is realizing to an increasing extent the importance of electrocardiography as a source of information about the action of the heart, but he often lacks the ability to derive the fullest information from the electrocardiogram. As a result the accumulation of knowledge about the effects of anaesthesia on the heart is slow. But, just as the cardiologist will have to learn enough of anaesthesia to understand its relation to his field, and there are many obvious problems linking these two, so will the anaesthetist have to learn enough about cardiology and the electrocardiogram to predict, observe and minimize the harmful effects of his anaesthetics on the heart. This he must be able to do since the need arises in the operating theatre and other places where an expert colleague may not be available for advice.

Dr Rollason sets out to satisfy this need. His book is written by an anaesthetist for anaesthetists. The author does not aim to make his anaesthetist colleagues electrocardiographic experts, nor to displace or disdain the true expert in that field. He does, however, present a simple but accurate introduction to electrocardiography with particular reference to the electrical changes in the heart which occur in the special circumstances of modern anaesthesia. His own studies and contributions concerning electrocardiography during anaesthesia have been considerable. He speaks therefore not only as an anaesthetist, sensitive to the needs of his colleagues, but as one with some claim to expert knowledge of electrocardiography and its interpretation in anaesthesia.

His book will undoubtedly encourage more anaesthetists to use modern physiological monitoring instruments and to learn how to interpret and make use of the information they provide. In time these instruments will be accepted by all as essential aids to safe anaesthesia. Electrocardiography is without question one of the important major examples. In adopting this view and practice, anaesthetists will, while not lessening the content of art, increase enormously that of science, in anaesthesia.

WILLIAM W. MUSHIN
M.A. M.B. B.S. F.F.A.R.C.S.
(HON.)F.F.A.R.A.C.S. F.F.A.R.C.S.I. F.F.A.(S.A.)
Professor of Anaesthetics,
Welsh National School of Medicine

PREFACE TO SECOND EDITION

In this edition an endeavour has been made to incorporate both the developments which have taken place during the past 5 years and the suggestions which were made by the various reviewers of the first edition.

Some of the chapters have been rewritten and two short chapters one on the ECG and Intensive Care, and the other on the ECG in Anaesthetic Research have been added.

Some illustrations have been deleted while others have been added. For the additional ones my thanks are due to Mr D.P. Hammersley and his staff and to my son Anthony N. Rollason.

I wish to express again my sincere thanks and appreciation of the considerable help I have received from my friend Mr J. M. Hough, M.A. in producing this edition.

I am also grateful to Dr D.S.Short for his helpful suggestions, to Mrs N.Taylor, Mrs A.Gibb, Mrs S.Pyper and Miss J.Leith for secretarial assistance and to Blackwell Scientific Publications for the efficient and courteous way in which they have produced both editions.

W. N. ROLLASON

Aberdeen
February 1968

PREFACE TO FIRST EDITION

During the past decade the ECG has established itself as an important ancillary aid to the anaesthetist not only during surgery and anaesthesia, under the peculiar conditions of the operating theatre, but also in the pre- and post-operative periods. This aid, however, is only of value if the anaesthetist is capable of interpreting the significance of the changes it portrays.

While there are a number of standard works on electrocardiography, both introductory and comprehensive, available for study, they do not present the subject from the point of view of the anaesthetist, and it is hoped that this small volume may help to remedy this defect. In presenting it an endeavour has been made to steer between the Scylla of over-simplification and inadequate presentation on the one hand, and the Charybdis of complexity and lack of clarity on the other. It is however in no way intended to supplant any of the existing works on the subject, but rather to complement them.

I wish to extend my sincere thanks and appreciation to Dr D. S. Short and Mr J. M. Hough, M.A. who reviewed the manuscript and offered many helpful suggestions, which have been incorporated. I am also grateful to Mr Hough for his assistance in writing chapter VI. My grateful thanks are also due to Mr W. Topp for all the reproductions, to my secretary Mrs A. H. Dickson for her unstinting help, and to Professor W. W. Mushin for his generous foreword.

W. N. ROLLASON

Aberdeen
September 1963

ACKNOWLEDGMENTS

I am grateful to the following authors and publishers for permission to reproduce the illustrations indicated:

Dr B.S.Lipman and Year Book Medical Publishers Inc., Chicago for Figs. 1, 19, 29, 32, 36, 43, 44, 62, 65, 68, 69 (from *Clinical Unipolar Electrocardiography*, 4th edn.);

Dr G.E.Burch and Henry Kimpton, London for Figs. 6, 27, 28 (from *A Primer of Electrocardiography*);

Dr L.Schamroth and Blackwell Scientific Publications, Oxford for Figs. 10, 21, 90 (from *An Introduction to Electrocardiography*);

Dr J.E.F.Riseman and the Macmillan Company, New York for Figs. 12a, b, c, 18 (from *P.Q.R.S.T.*);

Professor Saul D. Larks and Charles C. Thomas, Springfield, Illinois for Fig. 20 (from *Fetal Electrocardiography*);

Dr S.R.Arbeit and F.A.Davis Company, Philadelphia for Figs. 22, 25, 26, 33, 35, 37, 40, 45, 47, 56, 63 (from *Differential Diagnosis of the Electrocardiogram*);

Dr W.D.Wylie and Lloyd-Luke Ltd., London for Figs. 31, 82 (from *A Practice of Anaesthesia*);

Professor C.A.Keele and Professor Eric Neil and Oxford Medical Publications for Figs. 11, 13, 17 (from *Samson Wright's Applied Physiology*, 10th end.).

I would also like to express my thanks to:

Dr Milton Kissin and the Editor of the *American Heart Journal* for Fig. 5;

Dr K.Lupprian, Dr H.Churchill-Davidson and the editor of *The British Medical Journal*, for Fig. 64;

Dr M.Johnstone and the editor of the *British Journal of Anaesthesia* for Figs. 71–74;

Dr J.H.Cannard and the editor of *Anesthesiology* for Figs. 85, 87;

Dr J.G.Mudd and the editor of the *American Heart Journal* for Figs. 84(A), (B);

Dr C.F.Scurr and the editor of the *Proceedings of the Royal Society of Medicine*, for Fig. 81;

Dr D.Benazon and the editor of *Anaesthesia* for Fig. 83;

Dr J.L.Eiseman and the editor of the *American Journal of Surgery* for Fig. 98.

My thanks are also due to:

Dr D.S.Short for Figs. 42, 66;
Dr J.Cox for Fig. 86;
Dr C.C.Richards for Fig. 89;
Cardiac Recorders Ltd for Figs. 94(A) and (B), 95;
Dr C.R.Dundas for Figs. 97(A) and (C).

CHAPTER 1

INTRODUCTION

The heart muscle is unique among the muscles of the body in that it possesses the quality of automatic rhythmic contractions. These contractions produce weak electrical currents which spread through the entire body as the latter behaves like a volume conductor. The existence of these currents has been known for over a century. As early as 1856, Kölliker and Müller placed a frog's nerve muscle preparation in contact with a beating heart and were able to demonstrate twitches of the frog's muscles with each contraction of the ventricle. That these currents were measurable was demonstrated by Waller in 1887. He experimented with the capillary electrometer devised by Lippman in 1872 (Burch & De Pasquale 1964) and recorded the electromotive force from the precordium. But it was not until 1901, when Einthoven invented his string galvanometer that the current from the human heart-beat was registered in an accurate quantitative manner (Einthoven 1903).

While the first complete Cambridge electrocardiograph was supplied to Sir Thomas Lewis in 1911, it was not until 1918 that the human E.C.G. was studied during anaesthesia (Krumbhaar 1918; Heard & Strauss 1918).

It is known that the electric impulse in the normal heart originates in the sino-atrial node and travels through both atria to reach the atrioventricular node. The excitation wave then passes to the bundle of His proceeding along its right and left branches to the Purkinge fibres in the ventricles. Activation of the ventricular musculature takes place initially in the septum and subsequently in the free walls of both ventricles. It is primarily the electrical activity within the cardiac muscle which is recorded on the electrocardiogram. It does not record haemodynamic events, such as the efficiency or force of contraction of the myocardium. The major portion of the muscle mass consists of the free walls of the right ventricle, the left ventricle and the septum. Similarly, the major portion of the completed electrocardiogram consists of the electrical activity present in the septum and the two ventricles.

A cell is said to be polarized in the resting state, meaning that an equal number of ionic charges of opposite polarity (negative and positive) is present on both sides of the cell membrane. The positively charged ions (cations) are distributed on the outer surface and the negatively charged ions (anions) within forming a series of dipoles.

Stimulation makes the cell membrane permeable to the flow of ions, so that a flow of current occurs. On stimulation, depolarization locally ensues, and this depolarized locus is propagated along the cell membrane, setting up a moving boundary of potential difference between the stimulated and the resting areas. At the head of the advancing locus of activity, where the depolarized muscles encounters the boundary of the resting polarized muscle, a series of doublets appear. A doublet consists of a positive and negative charge in close proximity to each other on the surface of the cell membrane and of equal magnitude. Stimulation of the resting muscle thus produces an advancing wave of activity represented by a series of doublets which are propagated along the cell membrane and form a moving boundary of potential difference and this phenomenon is recordable.

Such a potential difference must be present between two electrodes in order to record a deflection. If there is no difference in potential, as in a zone of completely active or completely inactive muscle, no electrocardiographic deflections will be recorded.

Each mechanical contraction is accompanied by two electrical processes, depolarization (activation) and repolarization (recovery). The advancing doublets are so orientated during depolarization that the positive ion precedes the negative ion, i.e., the head is positive and the tail negative. When the muscle has been completely depolarized, it is referred to as apolarized. Repolarization then occurs and the outside of the membrane recovers its resting charge. During this process of repolarization the doublet is reversed, i.e. the head is negative and the tail positive. This is illustrated in Fig. 1.

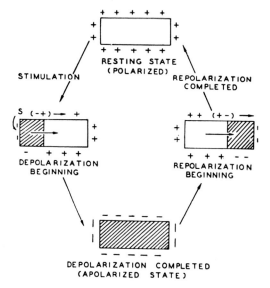

FIG. 1. Electrical activity associated with one contraction in a muscle fibre.

The electrocardiogram is the graphic representation of the electrical forces produced by the heart. Einthoven correlated the contracting heart with the electrocardiographic waves it produced and demonstrated that the P wave was related to the atrial contraction, whereas the QRS complex and the T wave were associated with the ventricular contraction. The waves produced by a normal cardiac contraction are shown in Fig. 2.

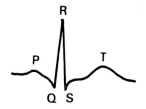

FIG. 2. Normal limb lead tracing.

CHAPTER II

THE NORMAL ECG

From the point of view of electric currents, the heart consists of two complex systems of cells, one constituting the atria and the other the ventricles, so that electrocardiographically, each system may be considered separately. Each mechanical contraction, atrial and ventricular, is associated with two electrical processes, i.e. depolarization and repolarization, illustrated in Fig. 1. Depolarization of the ventricles is represented by the QRS complex and repolarization by the T wave. The ST segment represents the period when all parts of the ventricles are in the depolarized or apolarized state. Depolarization of the atria is represented by the P wave; repolarization also occurs although the electrical record is usually obscured by the QRS complex, so that the T wave of the atrium—the Ta or Tp wave—is not normally seen. The atrial T wave (unlike that of the ventricle) is normally negative, i.e. below the base line. The base line is termed 'iso-electric'. The U wave is a wave low in magnitude following the T wave.

The PR and PQ interval, measured from the beginning of the P wave to the onset of the R or Q wave, respectively, marks the time which an impulse leaving the sinus node takes to reach the ventricles. The PR interval is normally not less than 0·12 second and not over 0·2 second.

The QRS interval measured from the beginning of the Q wave to the end of the S wave, represents the process of depolarization of the ventricles. During this time the cardiac impulse travels first through the interventricular system and then through the free walls of the ventricles. It normally varies from 0·05 to 0·10 second. The intrinsicoid deflection begins after the maximum QRS deflection has been inscribed i.e. at the peak of the R wave in QR complexes and at the lowest point of the S wave in the RS complexes. The

4

ventricular activation time—VAT—is the interval between the beginning of the QRS complex and the onset of the downstroke of the R wave which is known as the intrinsicoid deflection. The normal intervals are illustrated in Fig. 3.

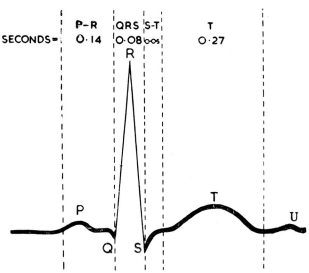

FIG. 3. Normal limb lead tracing illustrating the intervals.

The system is depolarized from the left to the right because a small branch of the left bundle of His is given off first. The subendo cardial regions of the ventricles are activated before the adjacent myocardial and subepicardial areas (Fig. 4).

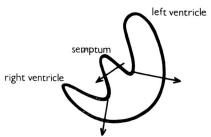

FIG. 4. Mechanism of ventricular depolarization.

The T wave represents repolarization of both ventricles. Hence one complete ventricular contraction (systole) is represented by the QT interval measured from the beginning of the Q wave to the

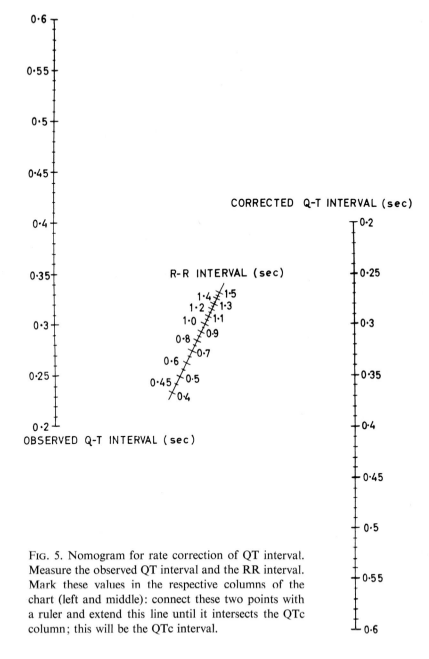

FIG. 5. Nomogram for rate correction of QT interval. Measure the observed QT interval and the RR interval. Mark these values in the respective columns of the chart (left and middle): connect these two points with a ruler and extend this line until it intersects the QTc column; this will be the QTc interval.

end of the T wave. This interval varies with age, sex and cardiac rate. When the rate is rapid, the interval is short and vice versa, e.g. at cardiac rates of 60–70 it is in the region of 0·4 second. The QTc interval is the QT interval corrected for cardiac rate from the formula $QTc=QT\sqrt{c}$ where c is the cycle length, which is 1 second when the pulse rate is 60 per minute and $QTc=QT$. It can be calculated for other pulse rates by means of a slide rule when the actual QT interval and cycle length are known. The QTc interval may also be obtained from the nomogram which is illustrated in Fig. 5.

Ventricular diastole extends from the end of the T wave to the beginning of the next Q wave.

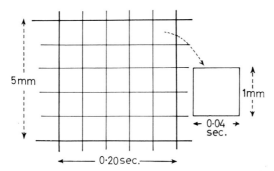

FIG. 6. Time markings and voltage lines of the electrocardiogram.

Horizontal and horizontal lines appear on all electrocardiograms. The horizontal lines represent time and are divided into larger and smaller squares. A large square indicates 0·2 second and a small square 0·04 second. The vertical lines represent voltage, 1 mm being equal to 0·1 mV, when the current is correctly standardized (Fig. 6).

To calculate the rate, the number of QRS complexes (for ventricular rate) or P waves (for atrial rate) occurring in a certain period of time are counted, e.g. the number of QRS complexes occurring in 3 seconds (15 large squares) is counted and multiplied by 20 to calculate the ventricular rate per minute. Some recording graphs have every fifteenth square marked by a vertical line at the upper border of the strip. Alternatively, the rule illustrated in Fig. 7 may

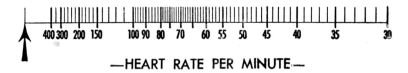

—HEART RATE PER MINUTE—

FIG. 7. The arrow should be placed on a heart complex (P or QRS) and the rate is obtained when the scale intersects the same portion of a complex two cycles removed. (Applicable for regular rhythm only).

be used. When the tracings are displayed on an ECG monitor, a videometer may be employed. This is hand operated and will record a reading of heart rate within a range of 40 to 160 per minute. It is illustrated in Fig. 8 and its method of use in Fig. 9.

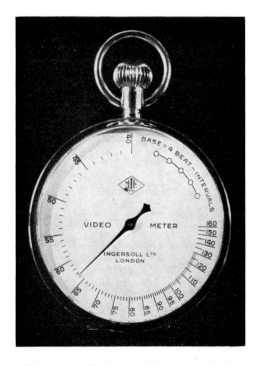

FIG. 8. The videometer. This is wound in an anticlockwise direction. By depressing the single control it will start, stop or zero the pointer sequentially.

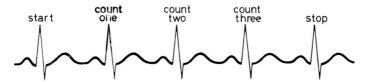

count one · count two · count three

start · stop

FIG. 9. Assuming the operator is viewing an ECG tracing the control having been wound and the pointer zeroed, is pressed to start at the first observed tracing and the next three tracings counted. At the fourth tracing the control is pressed to stop as shown. The pointer will then be observed at the figure representing the rate per minute.

THE ECG LEADS

STANDARD LEADS

These were introduced by Einthoven at the beginning of the century and have been adopted as the standard leads throughout the world.

Two electrodes placed over different areas of the heart and connected to the galvanometer will pick up the electrical currents resulting from the potential difference between them. The resulting tracing is termed a lead. For example, if under the first electrode a wave of 0·2 mV, and under the second electrode a wave of 0·6 mV occur over the same period of time, then the two electrodes will record the difference between them, i.e. a wave of 0·4 mV. A bipolar lead, therefore, records all electrical events between the two terminals by revealing the changes of one electrode over and above the changes affecting the other. The final tracing of the ECG is thus a composite recording of both electrodes.

In standard lead I the terminals are placed on the right and left arms (RA and LA). In lead II, the terminals are placed on the right arm and left leg (RA and LF-F = foot) and in lead III the terminals are placed on the left arm and the left leg (LA and LF).

In the standard leads the P wave should be upright in lead I and usually in lead II, but may be inverted in lead III. It should not be more than 2·0 mm in height or 0·1 second in duration.

Q must be small in leads I and II, but may be deep in lead III.

R should be at least 5 mm high in any one of the three tracings and no higher than 15 mm in any lead.

The ST interval should not be displaced more than 1 mm above or below the isoelectric line.

The T wave should be upright in lead I and II, or possibly diphasic in II, but may be inverted in lead III. It should be at least 2 mm high in one of these leads.

UNIPOLAR LEADS (V LEADS)

The standard leads record the difference in electrical potential between two points on the body produced by the heart action. Often this voltage will show smaller changes than either of the potentials and so greater sensitivity would be obtained if the potential of a single electrode could be recorded; an even greater potential will be obtained if the exploring electrode is close to the heart. If the exploring electrode is on the chest it will be particularly sensitive to the electric potential in the nearest part of the heart.

If this single electrode potential (unipolar) is to be measured, it is necessary to have a reference electrode at a fixed potential. This is obtained by connecting together the three standard lead electrodes to form a central terminal (Fig. 10). Electric theory shows that this must yield a constant potential, and in electrocardiography

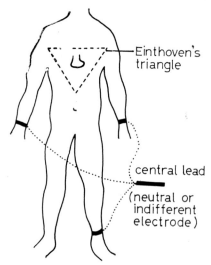

FIG. 10. Einthoven's triangle and the central terminal.

this is usually referred to as the Einthoven triangle (Fig. 10). It is usual to refer to the exploring electrode in this system as a V or 'voltage' lead. Two types of unipolar leads are employed: (a) limb leads, and (b) precordial leads.

(a) *Limb leads*. The potential value in the right arm may be obtained by connecting the exploring electrode to the right arm and the indifferent electrode to the other terminal of the galvanometer. This lead is termed VR. A similar technique is employed for obtaining the left arm and left leg extremity leads VL and VF respectively. The unipolar limb lead tracings are illustrated in Fig. 11.

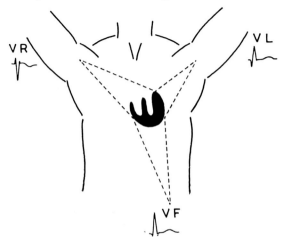

FIG. 11. The right arm lead faces the cavity of the ventricle, the left leg lead faces the inferior surface of the heart; this may be formed by the right or left ventricle or both, depending on the position of the heart. The left arm lead may face the cavity of the ventricles or the outside of the left ventricle, depending on the position of the heart. (Diagram by Dr D. S. Short.)

As the potential obtained by the exploring electrode of these leads is of low voltage the latter is usually augmented (A) by omitting the connection of the neutral terminal to the limb which is being tested. Thus the augmented unipolar limb leads are referred to as AVR, AVL and AVF respectively.

(b) *Precordial leads*. The second type of unipolar lead is a precordial lead and utilizes an exploring electrode to record the electrical potential of the right ventricle, septum and left ventricle. The unipolar chest leads are designated by the single capital letter 'V', followed by a subscript numeral which represents the location of the electrode on the precordium. Six chest positions are routinely used (V1–6):

V1: 4th intercostal space to right of sternum.

V2: „   „   „   „ left   „   „

V3: Midway between left sternal border and mid-clavicular line on a line joining positions 2 and 4.

V4: 5th intercostal space in mid-clavicular line.

V5: „   „   „   „ left anterior axillary line.

V6: „   „   „   „   „ mid-axilary line.

The position of the chest leads are illustrated in Fig. 12a, b and c.

C LEADS

In this type of lead, which like the standard lead is bipolar in character, the exploring C (chest) electrode is coupled with a relatively indifferent electrode placed either on the right arm (CR), left arm (CL), or left leg (CF). C leads are V leads minus the potentials in VR, VL and VF. As VR potentials are negative, their subtraction from V in CR records make all deflections more positive. This may be useful in demonstrating P waves of low voltage which may not be obvious in other leads; alternatively the P wave can be detected in an oesophageal or a S_5* lead, but these are not routinely employed. The behaviour of the P wave however assumes major importance in the diagnosis of an arrhythmia. The CL and CF leads are now rarely used.

The normal standard, augmented and precordial leads are illustrated in Fig. 13 and the C leads are compared with the standard leads in Fig. 14.

* S_5: For recording this lead the selector switch is set at lead I; the right-arm electrode is placed over the manubrium and the left-arm electrode over the right fifth interspace adjacent to the sternum.

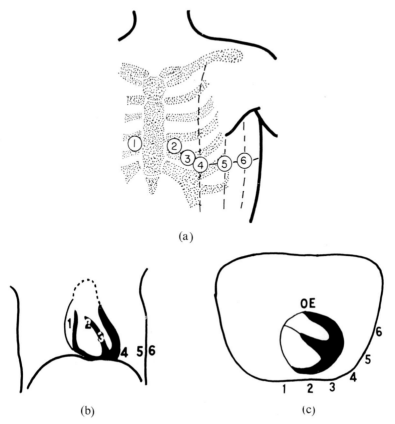

FIG. 12. (a) Position of the exploring electrodes on the precordium.
(b) The cardiac structures visualized by the precordial exploring electrodes.
(c) The cardiac structure visualized by both the precordial electrodes and the oesophageal electrode (OE).

ELECTRICAL ACTIVITY OF THE VENTRICLES

By convention, a wave is inscribed above the isoelectric line, i.e. positive when depolarization travels towards the exploring electrode from a remote area. It follows, therefore, that when an exploring electrode is placed over the right ventricle, it will receive an initial positive electrical impulse from septal depolarization (1), and a delayed negative impulse from left ventricular wall depolar-

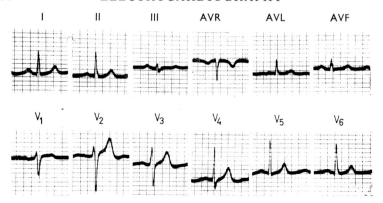

FIG. 13. Normal 12 lead ECG.

ization (2). The tracing of the right ventricular wall therefore is a RS complex as seen in Fig. 15.

Similarly, a left ventricular wall complex is composed of an initial negative septal current, and a later positive lateral wall current or a QR complex (Fig. 16).

Because of the relationship of the cardiac septum to the chest wall, the Q wave is not normally deep (1·5 mm or less). Therefore, as the exploring electrode is moved from the right ventricle over the chest to the left, the tracing evolves from the RS wave toward the QR complex. This progression from right to left is character-ized by a gradual elevation of the R as the S becomes more shallow, until R about equals the S in magnitude as the electrode overlies

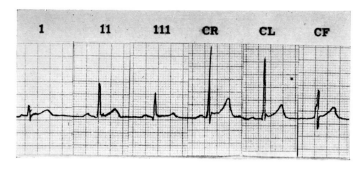

FIG. 14. Standard and C leads.

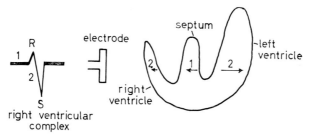

Fig. 15. The right ventricular complex.
(In the normal heart the larger left ventricular forces counteract and
in effect nullify the smaller forces of the right ventricle so that septal
depolarization (1) and left ventricular depolarization (2) need only be
considered.)

the septum. This is called the transitional zone. Farther left, S
becomes very small and in many tracings S will disappear and leave
the QR complex in position V6, thus completing the evolution.
These changes are illustrated in Fig. 17.

The smoothness of progression of the QRS complex is influenced
by a third factor besides the septal and lateral wall currents. This
is the positive tendency of endo-epicardial depolarization taking
place directly under the electrode. R in V5 and 6 may not be quite
as tall, because the heart recedes from the chest wall as the axilla is
approached. Moreover, reduction in voltage of R in V 1–3 may be
due in women to resistance of breast tissue. If R suddenly becomes
small in any position as observation is made from right to left,
disease is probably present.

The T wave in V 1 and 2 may be negative, but should be unalter-
ably upright beyond position 2 in adults.

The ST interval should normally vary between isoelectric and

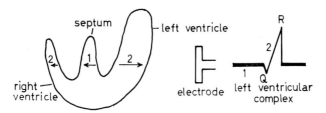

FIG. 16. The left ventricular complex.

2 mm. (Contrast with 1 mm in the standard leads.) The ST segment should never be more negative or higher than 2 mm.

Of less importance is the fact that R should not exceed 25 mm and that P, like T, may be negative in V 1 and 2.

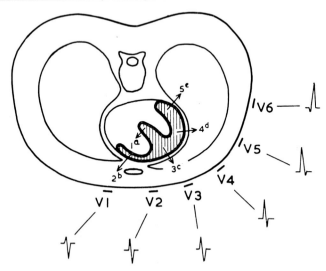

FIG. 17. Cross section through the chest to show the precordial leads and their relation to the heart; a, b, c, d and e show the order in which the electrical impulse spreads through the ventricle. Note the alteration in the configuration of the QRS complex between VI and V6. (Diagram by Dr D. S. Short.)

CLOCKWISE AND COUNTER-CLOCKWISE ROTATION OF THE HEART

The longitudinal axis of the heart runs obliquely from apex to the base of the heart. Rotation round this axis is conventionally viewed from below the heart looking towards the apex. This rotation is clockwise or counter-clockwise and either position can be normal.

In clockwise rotation the right ventricle assumes an anterior position and the precordial leads will record right ventricular or RS complexes in the V1–6 positions.

In counter-clockwise rotation the left ventricle will rotate anteriorly so that now both right and left ventricles assume an anterior position and QR complexes may be seen in the V4–6 positions.

ELECTRICAL AXIS OF THE HEART

Each ECG lead has a negative and a positive pole, and the location of these poles is referred to as the polarity of the lead. The line joining the poles of a lead is called the axis of the lead. The lead axis is orientated in a certain direction depending upon the location of the positive and negative electrodes. By convention the positive pole for lead I is to the left arm and the positive poles for leads II and III to the left leg. In the case of the unipolar limb leads, the positive pole is on one of the limbs and the negative pole is at zero potential.

The electrical intensity recorded by an electrode diminishes rapidly when the electrode is moved a short distance from the heart but less and less as the electrode is moved further away from the heart and with distances greater than 15 cm from the heart electrodes, in an electrical sense, may be considered to be equidistant from the heart.

The process of depolarization spreads from one region of the heart to the other in the form of an advancing wave front. The general, average or dominant direction of this wave front is known as the mean electrical axis of the heart and will be discussed further in Chapter III.

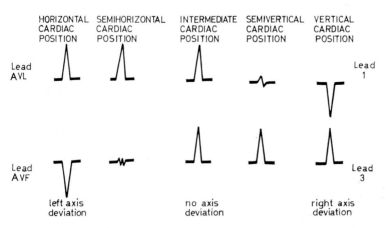

FIG. 18. The five patterns in the unipolar limb leads which indicate the cardiac position compared with the three patterns in the standard leads indicating axis deviation (Chapter III).

c

When the process of depolarization spreads towards a positive electrode an upward deflection is produced in the lead and when it spreads away from the positive electrode, i.e. towards the negative electrode, a downward deflection is produced in the tracing. When the electrical axis is normal the major deflections in both leads I and III are upright (Fig. 18).

ELECTRICAL POSITION OF THE HEART

Variations in the anatomical position of the heart are reflected electrically by the ECG.

In the neutral position, the anterior cardiac surface is largely right ventricle, and the apex and left border are composed of left ventricular wall. When the heart becomes horizontal it rotates round its antero-posterior axis which runs through the centre of the septum from the anterior to the posterior surface so that the left ventricle faces the left shoulder, and the right ventricle faces the left foot. Therefore, AVL (left arm) resembles the QR or left ventricular complex and AVF (left foot), the RS or right ventricular complex.

When the heart becomes vertical, the opposite event occurs and AVL tends to the RS right ventricular complex and AVF toward a QR left ventricular complex. In determining the position of the heart it is advisable to base the findings only on the location of the QR complex. When the heart occupies a neutral or intermediate position, the complexes of AVL and AVF tend to be the same, either the RS or the QR pattern. The positions of the heart and associated axis changes (see Chapter III) are illustrated diagrammatically in Fig. 18.

The AVR complex rarely enters the field of interpretation of the electrical position of the heart. Normally the AVR active electrode always faces some aspect of the cavity of the heart. The septal current runs mostly or entirely perpendicular to the electrode and causes either a small or no deflection at all. The lateral ventricular wall, however, produces a negative complex because depolarization travels away from the electrode which faces the cavity. In short, AVR normally is negative.

As the electrode is moved more posteriorly, it faces not only part

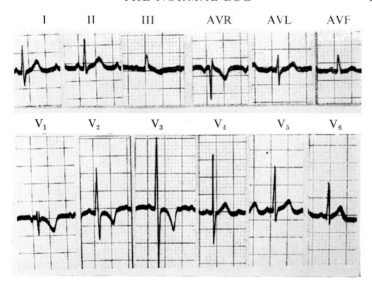

FIG. 19. Normal ECG in boy aged 2. Note the inverted T waves in V1, V2 and V3 which are normal at this age.

of the ventricular orifices or cavity, but also the posterior wall itself. The electrode is still perpendicular to the septum and no septal current occurs and the cavity still produces a negative wave. The posterior wall current, however, just over the electrode proceeds as usual from endocardium to epicardium and therefore towards this posterior electrode. A late positive wave results. The complex for the posterior wall of the heart is thus a deep QR. This deep cavity Q must not be confused with the shallow septal Q.

NORMAL VARIANTS OF THE ADULT PATTERN

Up to the time of birth, the foetal heart has had to provide a circulation through both the body tissues and the placental mass. The additional load is, by virtue of the patent ductus, shared between the right and left ventricles. As a result, at birth the development of the two ventricles is approximately equal, i.e. their wall thickness is similar. As a consequence, the ECG pattern simulates that of right ventricular hypertrophy in the adult (see Chapter III). This is associated with tall R waves and inverted T waves in the right precordial leads and is illustrated in Fig. 19.

In children, the tall R waves in the right precordial leads usually disappear after the age of five, but inverted T waves in the precordial leads frequently persist into the second decade.

In negroes this 'juvenile pattern' of T wave inversion in the precordial leads may persist into the third decade of life.

In older children, as in adults, an inverted T wave is common in V1. In the precordial leads, a negative T wave with a positive T wave in a position to the right of it is considered abnormal, so for a proper interpretation of the juvenile ECG leads V1-6 should be examined.

The child's heart is usually in the vertical position and only rarely in the horizontal position.

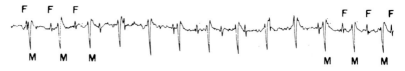

FIG. 20. The foetal complexes (F) can be distinguished from the maternal complexes (M).

THE FOETAL ECG

Much work has been done on foetal electrocardiography (Larks 1961; Kendal *et al* 1962; Hon 1965) and a recent comprehensive review (Shenker 1966) stresses the value of the ECG as a research tool in investigating placental function and the effect of drugs. There is, however, a need for the normal foetal ECG to be classified.

The maternal ECG is also present in the tracing when it is obtained from the mother's abdomen, but can usually be distinguished by a difference in amplitude and frequency (Fig. 20). The maternal ECG can, however, be eliminated when it is possible to place one lead on the foetal scalp and the indifferent electrode in the vagina.

VECTORCARDIOGRAPHY

At any instance the electrical activity of the heart may be described by a dipole which changes in magnitude and direction throughout a cardiac cycle. The normal ECG leads all measure the potential occurring at either one point (unipolar leads) or between two points (bipolar leads, e.g. standard leads). Vectorcardiography attempts to register either a two-dimensional projection of the dipole or the full three-dimensional dipoles. It is clear that a vectorcardiogram presents a more complete visualisation of the electrical activity of the heart than the standard leads (actually the simultaneous registration of two standard leads contains as much data as a vectorcardiogram obtained from the same leads). It is fairly simple to display a vectorcardiogram on an ECG monitor, but more difficult to obtain a permanent record.

There is little evidence of the use of this technique by anaesthetists and a recent text-book on heart diseases (Friedberg, 1966) states: 'The clinical usefulness of the oscilloscope vectorcardiograph is as yet hampered by its costliness, its cumbersome size, and the necessary skill required in its use. Furthermore, extensive studies are still needed to correlate pathological with vectorcardiographic findings'. Further discussion of this technique is not within the scope of this book; those interested in the subject should peruse *Clinical Vectorcardiography* by Chou and Helm (1967).

CHAPTER III

THE ABNORMAL ECG

Abnormal patterns may be associated with changes in the configuration of the P wave, QRS complex, ST segment, T and U waves, or by alteration in the PR, QRS and QT intervals. In addition, there may be disorders of cardiac rhythm. These abnormal patterns may be due to pathological states, but on occasion they may be due to artefact.

ALTERATIONS IN THE P WAVE

The P wave is tall and sharp, the height ranging from 2 to 5 mm in the right atrial hypertrophy, e.g. in pulmonary stenosis, and is referred to as P pulmonale.

It is usually bifid and conspicuously widened, the duration being in the region 0·12 second, in left atrial hypertrophy, e.g. in mitral stenosis, and is referred to as P mitrale. It is often best seen in standard lead II and lead VI (Fig. 21).

Lead II   Lead V1

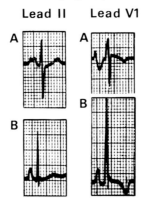

FIG. 21. ECG tracings showing the features of left and right atrial enlargement. A: Left atrial enlargement; B: right atrial enlargement.

It is widened and the voltage is low in hypertensive or aortic valve disease.

In lead I it is inverted in dextrocardia. This is illustrated in Fig. 22.

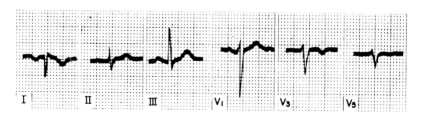

FIG. 22. Congenital Dextrocardia. Lead I is the mirror image of normal lead I; leads II and III are reversed and leads V3 and 5 resemble the right precordial leads.

It may be inverted in leads II and III in superior nodal (coronary sinus) rhythm (Fig. 48).

It may be inverted in leads I, II and III in inferior nodal rhythm.

It may be rendered unrecognizable by muscular tremors, such as shivering, so that determination of the site of the pace maker becomes impossible (Fig. 57). The configuration of the P wave frequently changes in height and direction when the pace maker shifts from the sinus node to varying portions of the atrium and the PR interval varies (Fig. 47). This phenomenon is called wandering pace maker and will be referred to again under ectopic rhythm.

ALTERATIONS MAINLY AFFECTING THE QRS COMPLEX

AXIS DEVIATION

In Fig. 23, the normal electrical cardiac axis is indicated by the arrow RA → LF, the length depending on the voltage. Its direction indicates an electrode link-up of right arm to left foot. This axis can be broken up into its horizontal or lead I (RA → LA) and vertical or lead III (LA → LF) vectors or components. Since a positive wave is inscribed when depolarization proceeds from

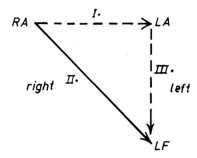

FIG. 23. The normal electrical cardiac axis.

RA to LF, then its two components, i.e. RA to LA to LF are similarly positive. Normal axis is seen in Fig. 13 (standard leads).

When the electrical axis of a heart shows left axis deviation of marked degree, the horizontal axis points not only towards the left shoulder but to a landmark above it. Such left axis deviation is illustrated in Fig. 24.

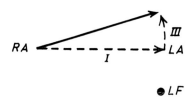

FIG. 24. Left axis deviation.

Lead I reveals positive depolarization from RA to LA, but lead III indicates a negative wave, in that depolarization travels from LA away from LF. Left axis deviation, therefore, manifests itself in a large R possibly with a small Q (left ventricular pattern) in lead I, and a negative complex or small R, and very deep S (right ventricular pattern) in lead III. This is illustrated in Fig. 25.

In marked right axis deviation, the electrical axis points to the right of the vertical, and therefore, the QRS complex in lead I is negative (from LA to RA) and that in lead III is positive (Fig. 26).

Negativity is produced by the S wave. If it were produced by the Q wave it would imply not axis deviation but infarction.

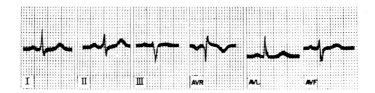

FIG. 25. Left axis deviation (leads I and III). Horizontal heart (leads AVL and AVF).

As leads I and III are the vectors of lead II, the waves in lead II are almost an addition to the other two leads.

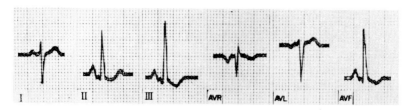

FIG. 26. Right axis deviation (leads I and III). Vertical heart (leads AVL and AVF).

Axis deviation may also be expressed in degrees (minus or plus, i.e. counter-clockwise or clockwise respectively), from the three o'clock axis (lead I line) of a triaxial system (Bayley 1943). Fig. 27

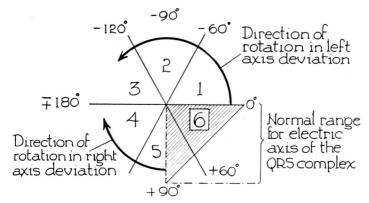

FIG. 27. The range of the normal axis of the QRS complex in degrees and the direction of rotation in left or right axis deviation.

illustrates the three types of axis deviation for the QRS complex, i.e. (1) normal axis deviation when the axis is between 0 and +90°, (2) right axis deviation when the axis is more positive than 90° and (3) left axis deviation when the axis is more negative than 0°.

Axis deviation may be obtained from a calculator (Rumball 1963; Milledge 1965) or from Dieuaide's chart (Fig. 28). It may also be calculated from the formula

$$\tan V = \frac{\frac{l_3}{l_1} + \frac{1}{2}}{0.866}$$

where V is the direction of the electric axis in degrees, l_1 is the electric vector in mm for lead I and is the algebraic sum of the R and S peaks in this lead, and l_3 is similarly the electric vector for lead III.

Some prefer to determine the mean electrical axis by the use of a hexaxial reference system (Schamroth 1966).

The direction of the mean normal electrical axis varies considerably with the age of the subject. In the infant under 6 months of age, the axis is greatly to the right (+130°). Between the ages of one and five years, the axis moves to the left, the average for these ages inclusive being about +52°. The axis then returns to the right at puberty, the average axis being about +67°. It again returns to the left in the adult, averaging about +58°. These changes in position are due mainly to the changing position of the heart in the thorax, except in the case of the infant.

Left axis deviation is present in (1) 10 per cent of normal people who are usually hypersthenic subjects, (2) left ventricular hypertrophy and dilatation, (3) left bundle branch block. Significant left axis deviation (−30° to −120°) is due to an intraventricular conduction defect involving the anterior-superior division of the left bundle branch (Davies and Evans 1960), (4) cardiac displacement to the left e.g. due to scoliosis, elevation of the diaphragm as a result of pregnancy, obesity or ascites. It is associated with such diseases as aortic stenosis or incompetence, hypertension, mitral incompetence, coarctation of the aorta, arterio-venous aneurysm and ostium primum defect.

LEAD Ⅲ

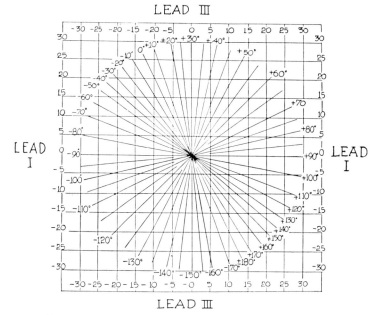

LEAD Ⅲ

FIG. 28. Dieuaide's chart for finding electric axis. To determine the electric axis of the QRS complex: the algebraic sum of the positive and negative deflections of the QRS complex in lead I is plotted along the lead I line (ordinate) and the algebraic sum of the positive and negative deflections of the QRS complex in lead III is plotted along the lead III line (abscissa). Perpendicular lines are drawn to these points. The point of junction of these perpendiculars represents the tip of the arrowhead of a vector force of the QRS axis, the tail being at zero or centre of the graph. The angle can be determined by the angle lines of the graph nearest the vector formed.

Right axis deviation is present in (1) the newborn (2) 10 per cent of normal children over the age of 8 years (3) right ventricular hypertrophy and dilatation (4) right bundle branch block and (5) cardiac displacement to the right. It is associated with such diseases as emphysema, mitral and pulmonary stenosis, and ostium secundum defect.

VOLTAGE CHANGES

An excessively high or low voltage of the QRS complex may be due to a standardization error and this should be checked. On the other hand it may be related to the thickness of the chest wall and to disease.

High voltage may be seen in patients with (1) a thin chest wall (2) ventricular hypertrophy and (3) hyperthyroidism.

Low voltage may be seen in patients with (1) a thick chest wall (2) a pericardial effusion, anasarca, myocarditis or myopathy (3) myxoedema (4) carbon monoxide poisoning and (5) emphysema.

In order to distinguish between axis and voltage changes of the RQS complex, the simultaneous observation of at least two of the standard leads is necessary (Rollason & Hough 1957a).

LEFT VENTRICULAR HYPERTROPHY

This is classically seen in patients with hypertension and is associated with left axis deviation. The diagnostic electrocardiographic signs are:—

(1) The R wave is likely to exceed 15 mm in one of the standard leads because of the generation of excess voltage.

(2) The tall R wave is followed by an inverted T wave. When the myocardium is severely hypertrophied or 'strained' it has been conjectured that the wave of repolarization or T wave is so retarded in its progress through the affected myocardium that other areas set up their own wave of repolarization. Consequently, a reverse progression occurs which imparts to the tracing a negative T.

(3) There is a delay in the onset of the downstroke of the R wave (the intrinsicoid deflection) over the left ventricular leads. Almost all the voltage changes concerned with the R wave in the chest leads normally take place during the upstroke. The downstroke of the R merely represents the time it takes for the detector to return to zero with no electric current flowing. In heart strain, delay in depolarization results in voltage changes even during the downstroke, so that from the peak of the R down to the base line, a longer than normal time elapses. This downward stroke, as indicated above, is termed the intrinsicoid deflection, and ordinarily its measurement is not performed. When the intrinsicoid deflection

is slurred in the chest leads, however, the delay characteristic of hypertrophy is obvious without measurement.

The ventricular activation time (VAT) is the time taken for an impulse to traverse the myocardium from endocardial to epicardial surface and is reflected in the measurement of the time interval from the beginning of Q to the peak of R and is prolonged when the onset of the intrinsicoid deflection is delayed.

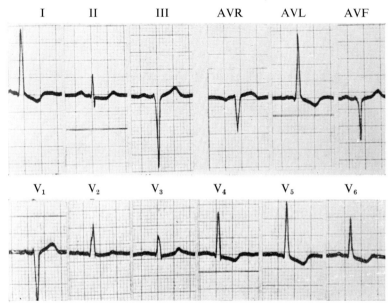

FIG. 29. Left ventricular hypertrophy ('strain pattern').

(4) In addition to the QRS and T wave changes the ST segment is frequently below the isoelectric line.

With left ventricular strain, high R and negative ST and T occur in left ventricular positions, i.e. V5 and V6, and this is illustrated in Fig. 29 and may be seen in hypertensive heart disease and aortic stenosis.

RIGHT VENTRICULAR HYPERTROPHY

This is usually associated with right axis deviation and the diagnostic electrocardiographic signs are:—

(1) Increased voltage of the R wave over the right ventricular

leads and altered R/S ratios, the S waves over the left precordial leads being greater than normal.

(2) A QR pattern may be present in lead AVR. This may be due to (a) marked clockwise rotation so that the left ventricle faces lead AVR or (b) the possibility that in right ventricular hypertrophy lead AVR faces a portion of the right ventricle and consequently faces the depolarization wave more directly. The diagnosis, of right ventricular hypertrophy, therefore, may be made when the QRS complex of AVR is more positive than negative, and about 50 per cent of all patients with an R as high as 4 mm have right ventricular strain, no matter how negative the Q or S may be. Moreover, a positive T in AVR is abnormal and may indicate right strain.

(3) Delayed onset of the intrinsicoid deflection over the right ventricular leads.

(4) Depression of the ST segment and inversion of the T wave over the right ventricular positions, i.e. V1 and V2, but here a normal negative T wave must be differentiated.

Right ventricular hypertrophy or 'strain' is illustrated in Fig. 30 and may seen be in pulmonary embolism and overtransfusion.

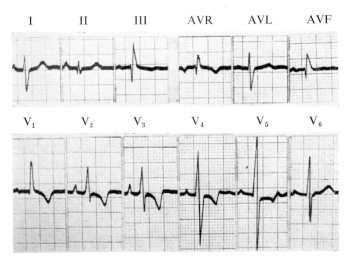

FIG. 30. Right ventricular hypertrophy ('strain pattern') P. pulmonale in leads V2 and 3.

Biventricular hypertrophy may occur, e.g. in ventricular septal defect, resulting in large amplitude diphasic QRS complexes in many leads. This is known as the Katz Wachtel phenomenon.

BUNDLE BRANCH BLOCK

This condition, which may be permanent, intermittent or transient, is due to a block in one of the branches of the bundle of His. When the QRS complex is 0·12 second or more, complete bundle branch block is present. If between 0·10 and 0·12 second, incomplete bundle branch block may be said to exist. Bundle branch block is primarily an electrocardiographic diagnosis and may occur in clinically normal hearts.

Bundle branch block is divided into right and left block. In typical block, the T wave is opposite to the main part of the QRS complex, but in atypical block the converse holds. Bundle branch block will be further discussed under disorders of cardiac rhythm.

ALTERATIONS MAINLY AFFECTING THE ST SEGMENT AND T WAVE

MYOCARDIAL INFARCTION

This probably results in three physiologically abnormal zones. The centre is the zone of necrosis (electrically inert), the surrounding area is the zone of injury (electro-negative), wherein either healing or necrosis will result, and around this is the zone of ischaemia. Healthy tissue is electro-positive. The necrotic centre affects the tracing in two major ways: (a) the R will be small or absent when the electrode subtends necrotic tissue, because depolarization is minimal or absent and (b) there will be a prominent, often wide, Q wave, because the dead tissue presents an open window to the electrode which is now electrically directly on the septum, or into the cavity of the heart.

The second, or zone of injury, causes the ST interval to be elevated if the electrode is directly over the area, or depressed if more remote resulting in a depressed or elevated base line respectively (Schamroth 1966).

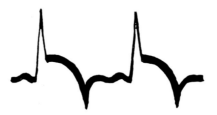

Fig. 31. The Pardee curve.

The classical 'Current of Injury' (the Pardee curve) is illustrated in Fig. 31 and it is on these raised ST segments that the diagnosis of infarction must be based.

The third or ischaemic zone causes inversion of the T wave.

Thus there are four changes: (1) small or absent R (2) deep Q (3) positive or negative ST and (4) inverted T.

A full thickness acute infarction of the anterior wall, presents all these changes in the precordial leads and this is shown in Fig. 32.

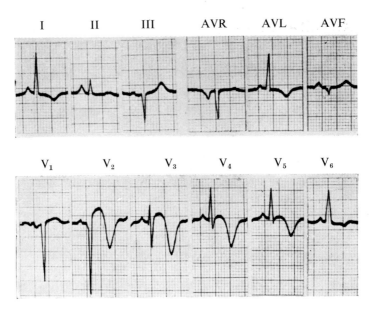

Fig. 32. Diffuse anterior myocardial infarction in a hypertensive patient.

Distinct alterations do not occur in posterior infarction because the active electrode is too remote, but depressed ST segments should make one investigate posterior infarction in the other leads, particularly leads II and III, AVF and the oesophageal lead. It should be suspected when there is a deep Q wave and an inverted T wave in leads II, III and AVF.

The right ventricle is very rarely involved.

Very low or absent R, elevated ST and depressed T over positions V5 and V6 indicate lateral wall infarction; over position V2 or V3 or possibly V1 also, septal infarction and over position AVL high antero-lateral infarction.

In old infarctions, the ST usually returns to the isoelectric base in a week or two, but the other changes remain for months or years.

In the standard leads, elevations of ST occur rapidly after anterior infarction in lead I. As the infarction becomes older, the ST descends towards the base line, but it carries the negative T with it in a characteristic equilimb curve likened to a bird in flight, the final part of the QRS complex going downwards into the initial segment of the negative T with a convexity directed upward. A Q in lead I occurs in anterior infarction, but the R is not too much affected. Thus a Q and a negative T in lead I, with an isoelectric ST indicates an older infarction. This is abbreviated as Q_1T_1.

Where Q_3T_3 occurs, posterior infarction is a possibility, but in lead III it may be a normal finding. If the ST segment is elevated more than 1 mm, a diagnosis of posterior infarction can be made, and if Q is wider than 0·04 second (1 mm), an old lesion exists in the presence of an isoelectric ST.

Usually old posterior infarction cannot be diagnosed positively from lead III or from the precordial leads, if Q is 0·03 second or less, as is most often the case. It is here that the unipolar augmented limb leads assist, because AVF in part faces the posterior heart. When AVF reveals an abnormal Q, there is strong presumptive evidence of posterior wall infarction whatever the standard leads show. Perhaps the most significance here is a Q longer than 0·04 second in AVF, whether or not it is deep.

Many infarcts do not show characteristic ECG changes; this is

D

particularly true of lateral infarcts in patients with hypertension. Moreover, in the case of minor or intramural infarctions the ECG may be normal.

In the interpretation of ST elevations or depressions, the ST segment is compared with the T–P interval following rather than with the PR portion of the base line preceding it. That part of the tracing between the end of the T wave and the beginning of the next P wave is considered the isoelectric level and forms the base line for determining displacement of the ST segment.

Elective surgery should not be undertaken for at least 3 months after a myocardial infarction (Fraser *et al* 1967).

Arrhythmia and conduction defects are unusual in anterior infarction but commoner in posterior and lateral wall infarction.

Mortality is much higher when the infarct is transmural but the prognosis improves if the patient survives the first two weeks postinfarction.

PERICARDITIS

The ECG pattern of pericarditis which causes injury to the sub-epicardial surface of the heart is best observed in the precordial leads and is characterized by widespread elevation of the ST segments, which maintain their normal upward concavity, and the absence of abnormal Q waves. These do not appear since the injury

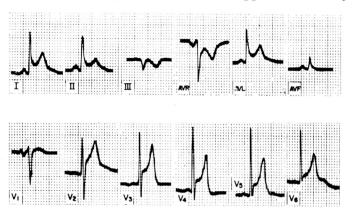

FIG. 33. Acute pericarditis pattern.

to the heart muscle is superficial. Inverted symmetrical T waves develop after the ST segment returns to the base line. Low voltage of the QRS complexes in all leads may also be observed and is due to the fact that the electrical currents in the heart are short-circuited through the pericardial fluid and thickened pericardium.

Fig. 33 illustrates the characteristic precordial lead pattern in acute diffuse pericarditis.

MYOCARDIAL ISCHAEMIA

This causes injury to the subendocardial surface of the heart and may cause bundle branch block particularly left bundle branch block and significant left axis deviation. An inverted U wave particularly when it develops after exercise always indicates myocardial ischaemia. The development of multifocal ventricular extrasystoles or post extrasystolic T and U wave changes are also important. More attention should be paid to evaluating the ECG changes after exercise when possible in the pre-operative assessment of the patient by the anaesthetist. These changes have been well tabulated by Schamroth (1966) but the classical changes are ST depression and T wave flattening or inversion in leads facing the surface of the heart whereas in leads facing the cavities (usually AVR) there will be a current of injury with raised ST segments.

During exercise muscle artefact may be eliminated by attaching the leads to chest and forehead, the resultant tracing resembles lead V4.

Myocardial ischaemia may be seen in the following conditions:

(1) arteriosclerosis of the coronary arteries, e.g. secondary to diabetes mellitus and myxoedema

(2) left ventricular hypertrophy

(3) aortic stenosis

(4) syphilitic aortitis

(5) pulmonary hypertension secondary to mitral stenosis or chronic diffuse pulmonary disease

(6) polycythaemia

(7) collagen diseases involving the coronary arteries, e.g. Buerger's disease

(8) anoxaemia, e.g. carbon monoxide poisoning
(9) hyperthyroidism
(10) rapid paroxysmal arrhythmias
(11) hypotension associated with severe haemorrhage
(12) hypotensive anaesthesia.
Myocardial ischaemia is illustrated in Fig. 34 and Fig. 78.

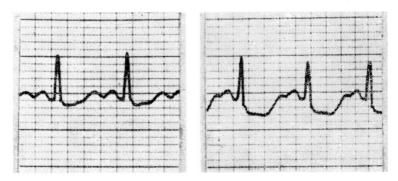

FIG. 34. Tracing on the left illustrates moderate and tracing on the right gross myocardial ischaemia (lead II).

ALTERATIONS IN THE U WAVE

Abnormal large U waves may be seen in hypokalaemia, during digitalis and quinidine therapy and in left ventricular hypertrophy, and inversion of the U wave may occur during myocardial infarction and/or ischaemia and in hyperkalaemia. Prominent U waves may also be associated with hyperventilation (Rollason and Parkes 1957).

Recently an X wave following U waves has been described during routine recordings of cases of cerebrovascular accidents and like the U wave is thought to indicate a very delayed completion of the process of repolarization (Agarwal and Gupta 1967).

DISORDERS OF RHYTHM

The ECG is most helpful and precise in detecting disorders of cardiac rhythm. These disorders may be physiological or pathological.

PHYSIOLOGICAL ARRHYTHMIAS

SINUS ARRHYTHMIA

This is usually associated with the two phases of respiration; during inspiration there is quickening of impulse formation in the SA node while during expiration there is a slowing.

Sinus arrhythmia is most frequently seen in children and young adults and is usually abolished by atropine and general anaesthesia, but it may reappear during controlled respiration. This arrhythmia is illustrated in Fig. 35.

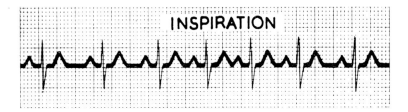

FIG. 35. Sinus arrhythmia.

SINUS TACHYCARDIA

This is associated with an increase in the rate of discharge of impulses from the SA node in the region of 100 to 160 beats per minute in the adult and is related to emotional disturbances or exercise. It may also be associated with disease such as anaemia, haemorrhage and hyperthyroidism and may occur in the ultra light planes of anaesthesia in the presence of painful stimuli. The T–P interval is usually abolished and it becomes necessary to use the PR or the PQ intervals for the isoelectric line.

SINUS BRADYCARDIA

In this condition the SA node discharges at a much slower rate in the region of 40 to 60 beats per minute and is characteristically seen in the highly trained athlete. Sinus bradycardia may also occur in disease such as myxoedema, obstructive jaundice, raised intracranial pressure and digitalis overdosage.

PATHOLOGICAL ARRHYTHMIAS

These may be classified as follows:

HEART BLOCK

    (1) Sino-atrial
    (2) Atrio-ventricular
        (a) 1st degree
        (b) 2nd ,,
        (c) 3rd ,,
    (3) Bundle branch block
    (4) Phasic aberrant ventricular conductions.

ECTOPIC RHYTHM

    (1) Extrasystoles
        (a) Atrial
        (b) Nodal
        (c) Ventricular
    (2) Paroxysmal tachycardia
        (a) Atrial
            (i) tachycardia
            (ii) flutter   S.V.T
            (iii) fibrillation
        (b) Nodal (unimportant)
        (c) Ventricular
            (i) tachycardia
            (ii) fibrillation
    (3) Escape beats

As far as the atrial arrhythmias are concerned Prinzmetal (1950) has shown that they depend upon the presence and behaviour of an irritable focus in atrial muscle. The type of arrhythmia produced depends on the rate of discharge of impulses from the ectopic focus. If the rate is slow, atrial extrasystoles result, but rates of 110 to 250 produce atrial tachycardia, rates of 260 to 340 atrial flutter, and rates of 400 to 600 atrial fibrillation. As the AV node can rarely transmit impulses faster than 210–20 per minute, physiological heart block results.

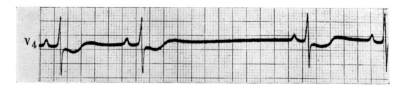

FIG. 36. Sino-atrial block. The PP interval that contains the pause is double the PP interval of the beats displaying normal sinus rhythm. A longer pause would indicate sinus arrest.

HEART BLOCK

This is a condition in which there is defective conduction in some part of the heart.

1. Sino-atrial block

Here the block is produced within the substance of the SA node, and the impulse has difficulty in getting out to activate the rest of the heart. It commonly results in the dropping of an entire PQRST complex. If alternate beats are dropped the heart rate is exactly half the normal. The condition is usually due to increased vagal tone acting on a susceptible SA node and can be abolished by intravenous atropine. Sino-atrial block is illustrated in Fig. 36.

2. Atrio-ventricular block

Here the whole bundle of His is damaged and changes occur in the following order:

(a) Delayed AV conduction. This is reflected in a prolongation of the PR interval which exceeds 0·2 second. This is referred to as first degree heart block and is illustrated in Fig. 37.

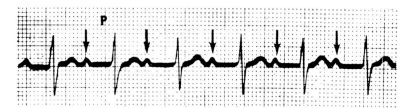

FIG. 37. First degree heart block.

(b) Failure of occasional and then of a larger proportion of the atrial impulses to reach the ventricles. The ventricles then respond to every second, third or fourth impulse from the SA node. This is referred to as second degree heart block.

A 2:1 heart block is illustrated in Fig. 38. Here the P waves are regularly spaced, but are twice as numerous as the ventricular impulses.

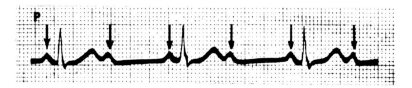

FIG. 38. Second degree (2 : 1) heart block.

Another form of second degree heart block is referred to as Wenckebach's phenomenon. The PR interval is usually normal at the onset of a cycle and gradually increases at each successive beat until the P wave is not conducted. This is illustrated in Fig. 39.

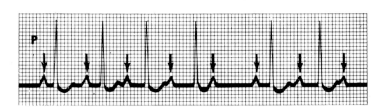

FIG. 39. Second degree heart block (Wenckebach's phenomenon).

First and second degree heart block is referred to as partial heart block.

(c) Complete or third degree AV block. Here none of the atrial impulses reach the ventricles and so the beats of atria and ventricles are completely dissociated, bearing no relationship whatever to one another. The ventricles beat with an independent rhythm, and at a slower rate—usually less than 40 per minute. The independent ventricular beats arise from the most rhythmic part of the ventricle, usually the region of the bundle below the site of the block. The excitation process, therefore, reaches the two ventricles along the normal channel of the two branches of the bundle. The ventricular complex is quite normal in character. This is illustrated in Fig. 40.

Complete or third degree AV block is a non-specific form of

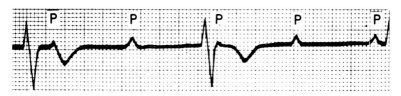

FIG. 40. Third degree (complete) heart block.

AV dissociation i.e. a rhythm where the atria and ventricles beat independently, the atria being activated by the sinus pace maker, and the ventricles by a nodal or ventricular pace maker, other forms of non-specific AV dissociation include ventricular extra-systoles and ventricular tachycardia.

AV dissociation in a specific sense refers to a rhythm known as interference dissociation. Here occasionally an impulse from the sinus pace maker reaches the AV node when it is not in a refractory state and produces an interference beat Fig. 41.)

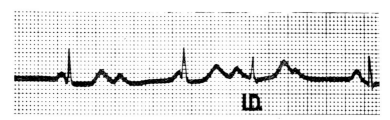

FIG. 41. Interference dissociation. I.D.: Interference beat (capture beat).

If the ventricular pace maker is located in the bundle branches or in the ventricular muscle (idioventricular rhythm), the QRS complexes are wide, slurred and notched, and have the character-istics of ventricular premature beats.

Widened and slurred QRS complexes may also, together with marked ST deviations and often absent P waves, constitute the tracing of the 'dying heart' (Fig. 42) which frequently precedes

asystole or ventricular fibrillation. These agonal ventricular complexes have been recorded up to 45 minutes after cessation of the
heart's contraction, and of respiration (Katz and Pick 1956).

Lead II

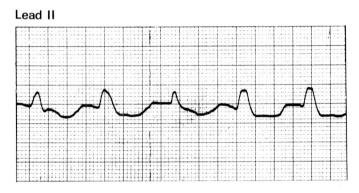

FIG. 42 'Dying heart' pattern.

3. *Bundle branch block*

This was referred to on page 31.

Right bundle branch block. When the right bundle is blocked, the
sequence of depolarization is:—

(1) Depolarization of the septum from left to right (the right side
is activated below the point of block by the stimulus from the left),
resulting in a R wave.

(2) Depolarization of the free wall of the left ventricle results in
a S wave.

(3) Depolarization of the free wall of the right ventricle resulting
in a R[1] wave. The electrical events on the left side of the heart are
normal.

The diagnostic electrocardiographic signs are:—

(1) QRS widened to 0·12 second or more

(2) Late onset of the intrinsicoid deflection over the right ventricular leads (V1 and V2)

(3) Increased amplitude of the R[1] wave in the right precordial
leads

(4) Depression of the ST segment and inversion of the T wave
(typical block) over the right precordial leads.

(5) Left ventricular precordial leads show a slurred broad S wave due to the late right ventricular depolarization

(6) A QR pattern in lead AVR

(7) Frequently a broad S wave in lead I

Right bundle branch block is illustrated in Fig. 43.

It is sometimes found in a heart which is otherwise normal. It then may have no serious significance.

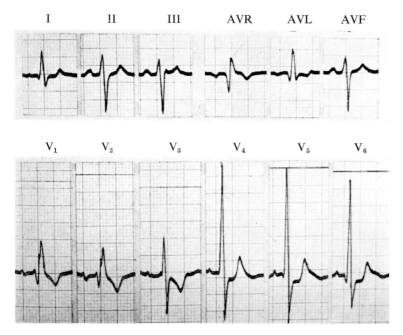

FIG. 43. Right bundle branch block (horizontal heart).

In disease, right bundle branch block is associated with conditions producing great dilatation of the right ventricle, such as atrial septal defects where it occurs in partial or complete form in 95 per cent of cases.

It may also be associated with pulmonary embolism, coronary artery, hypertensive and valvular heart disease.

Left bundle branch block. When the left bundle is blocked the sequence of depolarization is:—

(1) Depolarization of the septum is from right to left so that the left side of the septum below the point of the block is activated by the stimulus from the right

(2) Depolarization of the free wall of the right ventricle

(3) Depolarization of the free wall of the left ventricle. The electrical events in the right side of the heart are normal.

The diagnostic electrocardiographic signs are:—

(1) QRS widened to 0·12 second or more

(2) Late onset of the intrinsicoid deflection in leads over the left ventricle (V4–V6)

(3) Depressed ST segments and inverted T waves over the left chest leads.

(4) Right ventricular precordial leads show a slurred broad S wave due to the late left ventricular depolarization and the ST segments may be slightly elevated.

Left bundle branch block is illustrated in Fig. 44.

Very rarely left bundle branch block may be present in a clinically normal heart. It is seen most commonly in coronary artery disease, hypertensive heart disease and aortic stenosis.

Wolff-Parkinson-White syndrome. This is characterized by a wide QRS complex (0·11–0·14 second) and a short PR interval (0·10 second or less). This is illustrated in Fig. 45. The slurred and thickened proximal limb of the QRS complex is called the delta wave.

The syndrome usually occurs in healthy young persons who have a tendency to recurrent attacks of cardiac arrhythmia and in itself is not indicative of organic heart disease. It must be distinguished from bundle branch block. Although the PR interval is short the PS interval is normal.

4. *Phasic aberrant ventricular conduction*

An isolated, bizarre QRS complex is not necessarily the result of an ectopic ventricular discharge but may be due to a temporary bundle branch block following a supraventricular impulse and has been termed aberrant ventricular conduction. This phenomenon

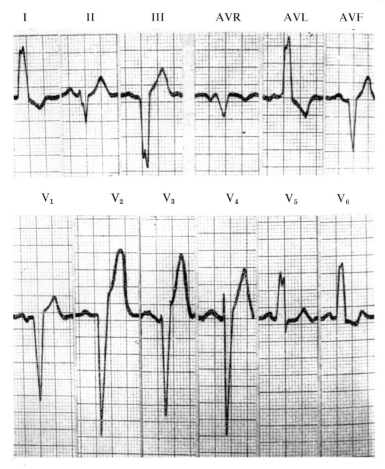

FIG. 44.   Left bundle branch block.

is due to unequal refractory periods of the bundle branches and may be temporary (phasic) or permanent (non-phasic) (Schamroth & Chester 1963). The recognition of this conduction defect is important as the differentiation of supraventricular from ventricular rhythms affects both prognosis and treatment. For the diagnosis of phasic aberrant ventricular conduction there must be a P wave before, and related to, the bizarre QRS complex. P waves are usually best seen in leads V1, CRI, an oesophageal, or S_5 lead.

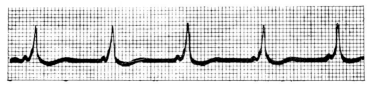

FIG. 45. Wolff-Parkinson-White Syndrome.

ECTOPIC RHYTHM

1. *Extrasystoles*

(a) *Atrial.* If the atrium is stimulated during diastole after its refractory period has passed, it responds with a premature contraction. An impulse is transmitted to the ventricles which contract too. The P wave is usually abnormal in configuration, (e.g. inverted or isoelectric) and the PR interval shortens, but the succeeding ventricular complex is usually normal. The next atrial impulse arising in the SA node appears after a pause equal to the normal diastolic period or a little in excess of it. An atrial extrasystole is illustrated in Fig. 46. When the atrial beat is so premature that the

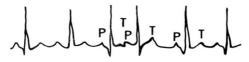

FIG. 46. Atrial extrasystole.

ventricles are in refractory state they fail to respond. Atrial extrasystoles are common during cardiac surgery and appear to have no special significance.

The phenomenon of wandering pacemaker refers to a shift in origin of the stimulus between the SA and AV nodes and is characterized by changes in the form of the P waves and by changing PR intervals from beat to beat in the same lead. It is sometimes referred to as a shifting or sliding nodal rhythm. Fig. 47 illustrates a wandering pacemaker with excursions limited between the SA and upper AV node and a wandering pacemaker in the AV node.

(b) *Nodal.* Here the P wave, which is usually deformed, is placed shortly before or after, or may coincide with a ventricular complex. The beat occurs prematurely and is followed by a compensatory pause. It can be precipitated by increased vagal activity.

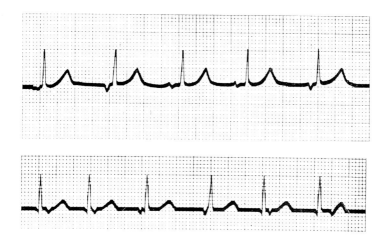

Fig. 47. *Upper tracing:* Wandering pacemaker with excursions limited between the SA and upper AV node.
Lower tracing: Wandering pacemaker in the AV node.

When the ectopic focus remains in the AV node, nodal rhythm is produced. There are three types of nodal rhythm depending on whether the impulse arises in the upper, mid or lower portion of the AV node. When the impulse arises in the upper portion of the node, the P wave falls just before the QRS complex and is referred to as superior nodal or coronary sinus rhythm. When the impulse arises in the mid portion of the node, the P wave is buried in the QRS complex and as a consequence is not visible. This is referred to as mid nodal or just nodal rhythm. When the impulse arises in the lower portion of the node, the P wave follows the QRS complex and is referred to as inferior nodal rhythm.

Nodal rhythm is frequently seen during anaesthesia and appears to have no special significance. It is usually associated with increased vagal tone. It may also occur during stimulation of the atrial musculature during surgery and during cardiac catheterization. Nodal rhythm is illustrated in Fig. 48.

(c) *Ventricular.* If the ventricle is stimulated during diastole after its refractory period has passed, it also responds with a premature contraction. The ventricular complex is abnormal and is

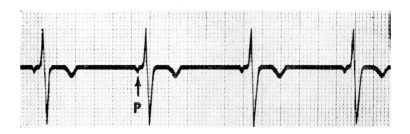

FIG. 48. Nodal rhythm.

not preceded by a P wave. The next P wave is usually 'buried' within this ventricular complex. The excitation process which arises in the new focus spreads radially over the surface of the ventricular muscle in all directions: it also penetrates the ventricular wall to reach the endocardium and so invades the Punkinje tissue which transmits the excitation process rapidly over its own side of the heart. The same change occurs later in the contralateral ventricle. As the time taken for the excitation process to affect the whole of both ventricles is prolonged, the QRS will exceed 0·12 second in duration; as the pattern of invasion is abnormal, the deflections of the QRS will be abnormal in appearance. The pattern of repolarization is also altered with consequent changes in the ST segment and the T wave. There is no isoelectric portion of the ST segment and the T wave takes off from a level above or below the isoelectric line and usually has a direction opposite to that of the main deflection of the QRS complex. A ventricular extrasystole is illustrated

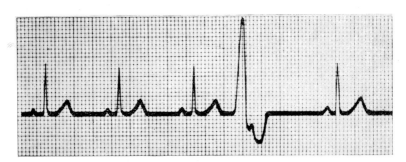

FIG. 49. Ventricular extrasystole.

in Fig. 49. When the ectopic focus originates in the right ventricle, the QRS deflection resembles a left bundle branch block pattern as seen in the right precordial leads and when it originates in the left ventricle the QRS resembles right bundle branch block pattern as seen in the right precordial leads. Ventricular extrasystoles tend to follow long R–R intervals and this is known as the 'Rule of Bigeminy'. The compensatory pause of the extrasystole provides another long R–R interval which tends to produce a further extrasystole so that the process may be self perpetuating resulting in bigeminal rhythm* (Fig. 70). If ventricular extrasystoles become frequent, they interfere with the efficiency of the circulation as the output produced by a premature beat is less than normal because the ventricle has not had time to fill. Multifocal ventricular extrasystoles (Fig. 50) are usually ominous and may be followed by ventricular fibrillation (Fig. 51).

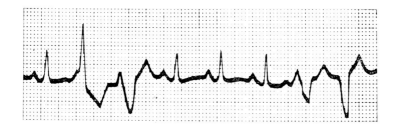

FIG. 50. Multifocal ventricular extrasystoles.

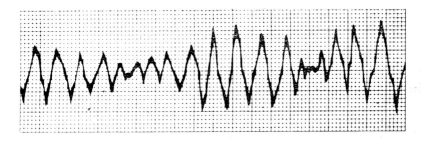

FIG. 51. Ventricular fibrillation.

* Bigeminal rhythm may also be caused by alternate atrial or nodal extrasystoles or by a 3 : 2 AV block.

E

2. *Paroxysmal tachycardia*

This term is applied to attacks of rapid heart action where ventricular contraction responds to regular impulses arising in a focus removed from the SA node, the rate may be as slow as 100 per minute or as rapid as 210 or even faster in infants. Three forms of paroxysmal tachycardia are recognized according to whether the ectopic focus of stimulus formation is situated in the atrium, AV node or ventricle. The essential characteristics of all types of tachycardia are:

    1. They begin suddenly
    2. The first beat is a premature one
    3. The beats are absolutely regular
    4. They terminate suddenly
    5. Carotid sinus pressure, pressure on the eyeball, or the administration of a vasopressor or neostigmine, may change the rate or stop the paroxysm completely.

(a) *Atrial*. (i) Atrial tachycardia. Here there is a rapid succession of abnormal P waves. The fact that the impulse initiating atrial contraction commences in a focus removed from the SA node explains the inversion or other deformity of the P wave. Often the P waves appear to be unaltered but when they are compared with those in a tracing obtained before or after the paroxysm, it will be seen that during the attack they differed from the normal for that individual. The ventricular complexes following the P wave are usually normal. Paroxysmal atrial tachycardia is illustrated in Fig. 52.

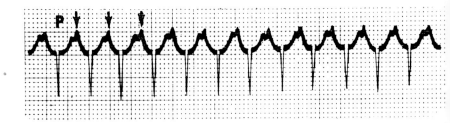

FIG. 52. Paroxysmal atrial tachycardia.

(ii) <u>Atrial flutter.</u> Here the P waves are absolutely regular in rhythm. They are characterized by a rapid upstroke and a more gradual downstroke and by the absence of any isoelectric interval between the waves. The waves occur in rapid succession, usually 260–340 per minute, but occasionally as much as 400 per minute. The ratio between atrial and ventricular complexes is commonly 2:1 as a physiological heart block occurs but the ventricle may respond less frequently so that a 4:1 response is not unusual. When the ratio is 1:1 the tracing is difficult to distinguish from one of paroxysmal atrial tachycardia, but in the latter condition the rate is usually less than 210. Fig. 53 illustrates a case of atrial flutter.

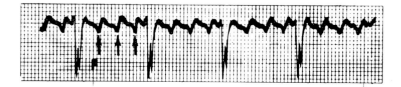

FIG. 53. Atrial flutter.

Digitalis often converts flutter to fibrillation and with the cessation of its administration a normal rhythm may result.

Atrial flutter may be precipitated by cardiac catheterization and other cardiac manoeuvres.

(iii) <u>Atrial fibrillation.</u> Here the tracing shows no true P waves which are replaced by oscillations called 'f' waves, which are irregular in shape, at a rate of 400–600 per minute. The ventricular complexes are usually normal but they occur at irregular intervals which is a characteristic feature giving rise to the typical irregular irregularity of the pulse. Exceptionally, the pulse may be slow and completely regular when complete heart block is associated with atrial fibrillation.

Atrial fibrillation is illustrated in Fig. 54.

This arrhythmia occurs most commonly in rheumatic mitral valvular disease, coronary artery disease and hyperthyroidism. It may also occur in clinically normal hearts and in association with

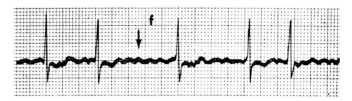

Fig. 54. Atrial fibrillation.

cardiotomy and hypothermia. Its onset may decrease cardiac output by as much as 40 per cent.

(b) *Nodal*. Here the P wave is usually inverted and the PR interval shortened. The P wave precedes or follows or, occasionally, coincides with the ventricular complex which is usually normal in configuration. Nodal tachycardia is illustrated in Fig. 55.

When the rate is rapid it is impossible to differentiate nodal from atrial tachycardia and in such instances the term supraventricular tachycardia is applied.

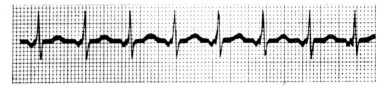

Fig. 55. Nodal tachycardia.

(c) *Ventricular*. (i) Ventricular tachycardia. Here the P waves are lost in the large excursions of the ventricular complexes which have a wide and notched appearance. They are regular in rhythm and are followed by large secondary T waves which are directed opposite to the main deflection of the QRS complex. Paroxysmal ventricular tachycardia is illustrated in Fig. 56.

This arrhythmia may precede ventricular fibrillation and it may occur after coronary occlusion.

(ii) Ventricular fibrillation. Ventricular fibrillation (Fig. 51) occurs when individual myocardial fibres are out of phase. Excitation then spreads from one fibre which contracts to another which is resting. This excitation is effective only when the refractory period is abnormally short.

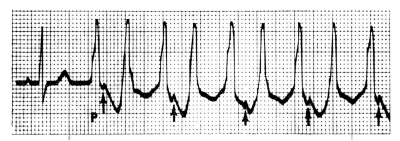

Fig. 56. Paroxysmal ventricular tachycardia.

Under normal conditions the long refractory period of cardiac muscle as compared with that of skeletal muscle protects it from fibrillation.

3. Escape beats

The SA node, ectopic atrial tissue, the AV node and the Purkinje cells of the ventricular musculature all have potential pace making properties but the fastest pace maker i.e. the SA node normally dominates the heart. If for some reason the dominant pace maker is suppressed a subsidiary pace maker can take over and initiate the cardiac impulse. This escape from the dominant pace maker constitutes a safety mechanism and prevents asystole. Escape is atrial when it originates in ectopic atrial tissue, nodal when in AV nodal tissue and ventricular when in ventricular tissue.

The average inherent discharge rate of the SA node is 76 per minute; the AV node 60 per minute; the bundle of His. 50 per minute, and the Purkinje cells of the ventricular muscle 30 per minute.

COMBINED MECHANISM

It should be realized that more than one arrhythmia may occur simultaneously as in the case instanced above, where atrial fibrillation occurs in the presence of complete AV block.

The management of cardiac arrhythmia during anaesthesia and analgesia has been discussed elsewhere. (Rollason, 1967b.)

Electrical Alternans

This does not cause a disturbance of rhythm but consists of an alternation in the amplitude of the QRS complexes. It is only significant when associated with a slow heart rate.

ARTEFACTS

These may be grouped into (a) those common to electrocardiography wherever it is performed, and (b) those peculiar to electrocardiography in the operating theatre.

(a) COMMON ARTEFACTS

(i) *Muscle tremor*. It is important for the conscious patient to be warm and relaxed when the record is taken as any muscle tremor such as that produced by shivering can alter the tracing. This type of interference is illustrated in Fig. 57.

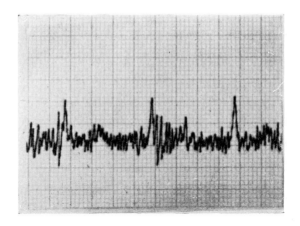

FIG. 57. Muscle tremor.

(ii) *Movement of the patient*. Movement on the part of the patient with the associated contraction of skeletal muscle causes sudden changes in the current conducted through the galvanometer resulting in sudden deflections. In addition, movement of the subject may disturb the contact of some electrodes on the body. These effects are illustrated in Fig. 58.

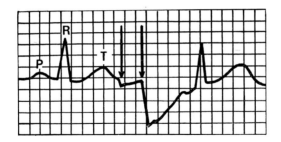

FIG. 58. Movement of the patient.

(iii) *Shifting of the base (isoelectric) line.* This is often due to cutaneous currents, polarization of the electrodes, variations in cutaneous resistance or wires conducting electricity in the vicinity of the recording leads and is illustrated in Fig. 59.

(iv) *Loose contacts.* These may occur in any part of the circuit and produce sudden shifting of the base line as shown in Fig. 60.

(v) *Inadequate earthing.* When the patient or the machine is not properly earthed alternating current may produce gross interference due to 50 cycle alternating current as shown in Fig. 61.

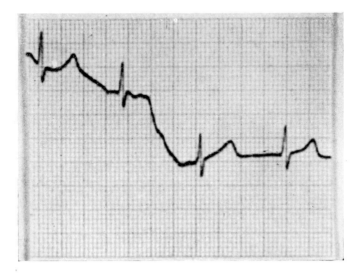

FIG. 59. Shifting of the base line ('Coney Island' ECG).

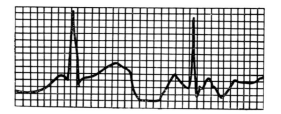

FIG. 60. Sudden shifting of the base line.

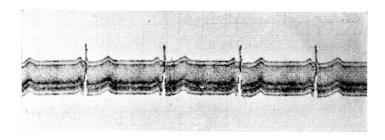

FIG. 61. 50 cycle interference ('hum').

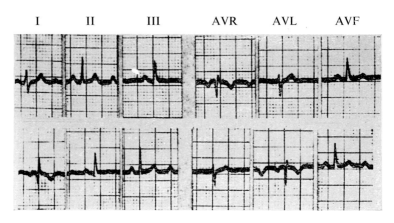

FIG. 62. *Upper tracing:* normal ECG picture.
   Lower tracing: Leads incorrectly connected. Right and left arm leads reversed. Lead I is mirror image of itself, leads II and III are reversed, as are also leads AVR and AVL. (Compare with Fig. 21 which illustrates the ECG in dextrocardia.)

(vi) *Incorrectly connected leads.* When abnormal wave forms for a particular lead are present incorrect placement of the leads should be suspected. For example, if the right and left arm leads are reversed, simulating dextrocardia, lead I becomes the mirror image of itself, and leads II and III become reversed as do also leads AVR and AVL. This is illustrated in Fig. 62.

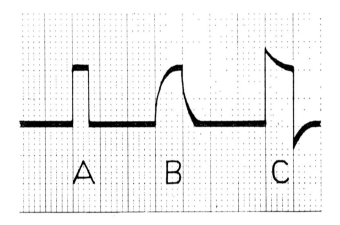

Fɪɢ. 63. (A) Correct standardization (B) overdamping (C) underdamping.

(vii) *Inaccurate calibration.* ECG machines provide an internal 1 mV potential for calibration. Pressing a switch a 1 mV deflection can be produced and adjustment of the gain control enables this deflection to be made exactly 1 cm. Incorrect calibration will cause the ECG voltages to appear either too large or too small and will lead to faulty interpretation. In addition, the shape of the voltage change on switching on or off will indicate whether the machine is functioning correctly. If the machine does not function satisfactorily on this test (Fig. 63) any ECG pattern recorded is liable to be distorted. The importance of frequent calibration cannot be overstressed.

The problem of artefact has been discussed by Bradlow (1964).

(b) ARTEFACTS PECULIAR TO THE OPERATING THEATRE
These will be discussed in Chapter V.

CHAPTER IV

THE EFFECT OF ANAESTHETIC AGENTS, ELECTROLYTE IMBALANCE AND CARDIAC DRUGS ON THE ECG

PREMEDICATION

Apart from the sinus tachycardia usually produced by such drugs as atropine and chlorpromazine, routine premedication appears to have no significant effect on the ECG in the healthy subject. As the main coronary inflow occurs in diastole, drugs which increase the heart rate shorten diastole and should be avoided in patients with hyperthyroidism and cardiac disease, except those with heart block.

Apprehension and anxiety are common causes of tachycardia and should be dealt with by appropriate reassurance and sedation. The barbiturates and tranquilisers appear to produce no significant ECG changes in normal dosage.

MORPHIA AND SCOPOLAMINE

Kurtz et al (1936) studied premedication with these agents and found a tendency to produce small changes in the QRS complex and T wave together with slight ST depression and an increase in pulse rate.

ATROPINE

In the conscious and fit patient intravenous atropine may produce a tachycardia or a bradycardia (Rollason 1957; Thomas 1965). Large doses accelerate and small doses slow the heart rate. Rapid injection tends to produce tachycardia and ECG changes (Gottlieb and Sweet 1963). A depression of the ST segment up to 1 mm. can, however, be produced by tachycardia alone. The drug may produce a supraventricular arrhythmia, such as nodal rhythm and nodal extra systoles (Averill and Lamb 1959; Jones *et al* 1961) and in the presence of adrenaline, CO_2 retention and electrolyte imbalance it may precipitate ventricular fibrillation. It may predispose to a multifocal ventricular arrhythmia in patients anaesthetised with cyclopropane and halothane and in patients subjected to topical analgesia with cocaine (Orr and Jones 1967).

There is evidence in the dog that it increases the oxygen consumption of the myocardium more than the coronary flow (Scott *et al* 1959).

It has been used preoperatively in a dose of 2 mg. intramuscularly to differentiate biliary from arteriosclerotic heart disease (Kaufman and Lubera 1967). Marked improvement in the ECG pattern followed in those patients with biliary disease.

It should however be appreciated that atropine is a potentially lethal drug and should only be given when specifically indicated.

Other drugs used in premedication such as pethidine, the antihistamines, the phenothiazines and the neuroleptic agents produce no significant ECG changes in normal dosage in the fit patient provided respiratory depression and CO_2 retention are avoided. Neuroleptanalgesia however does not protect the patient from reflexes which predispose to cardiac arrhythmia (Eerola *et al* 1963).

INDUCTION AGENTS

BARBITURATES

Thiopentone may cause an increase in the height of the P wave but this is probably related to an increase in pulse rate and a fall in BP rather than to the drug *per se* (Rollason and Hough 1958).

Pre-existing ventricular extra systoles may be abolished by both thiopentone and metho-hexitone.

While sinus tachycardia may occur during the ultra light methohexitone technique now frequently used in chair side dentistry it is unusual to observe any significant ECG changes except in the very nervous patient (Rollason and Dundas 1966).

PROPANIDID

This new intravenous induction agent is a eugenol derivative marketed under the name of Epontol. Apart from an occasional sinus tachycardia no significant ECG changes have so far been observed when the drug is injected slowly (Wynands and Burfoot 1965; Rollason 1967a). Changes however have been recorded when the drug is injected more rapidly and a brief anti-arrhythmic action has been demonstrated (Johnstone and Barron 1968).

DIAZEPAM

This benzodiazepine derivative is marketed under the name of Valium and while it has been widely used as a psychotherapeutic agent by psychiatrists it has only relatively recently been used as an intravenous induction agent by anaesthetists. So far no significant ECG changes have been observed (McClish 1966) although the occasional vagotonic reaction has been observed when used in the high dosage necessary to induce unconsciousness in the unpremedicated patient (Rollason 1968b).

GAMMA-HYDROXYBUTYRATE

This new intravenous agent has yet to be proved. Induction is slow and may be accompanied by extrapyramidal movement. Its duration of action is prolonged and, furthermore, recovery may be associated with emergence delirium. It is accordingly unsatisfactory as a sole agent. So far the only recorded ECG change has been a sinus bradycardia during induction (Solway and Sadove 1965), but this does not occur when no other drug has been given beforehand.

MUSCLE RELAXANTS

Apart from the sinus tachycardia produced by gallamine triethiodide and the hypotension which sometimes follows the administration of d-tubocurarine suxamethonium appears to be the only relaxant which produces significant ECG changes in the absence of hypoxia and CO_2 retention.

The more recently introduced non-depolarising relaxants, Alloferin (diallyl-nortoxiferine) and pancuronium bromide are reputed to be devoid of cardiovascular side effects although the latter agent which is a steroid compound has yet to be fully assessed. So far no ECG changes have been observed.

SUXAMETHONIUM

This relaxant when given intravenously can not only produce a bradycardia but also a disturbance of rhythm in both children and adults. The nature of the arrhythmia is a depression of excitation and conduction of the cardiac impulse producing changes in the P wave, PR interval, QRS complex and asystole lasting up to 16 seconds (Martin 1958; Lupprian and Churchill-Davidson 1960; Sagarminaga and Wynands 1963). These changes are illustrated in Fig. 64.

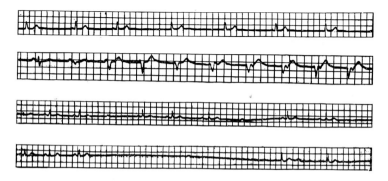

FIG. 64. *Top tracing:* Variations of the P wave; *Second tracing:* Wide QRS complexes followed by inverted P waves; *Third tracing:* Wenckebach's phenomenon; *Bottom tracing:* Ventricular standstill.

A case of prolonged cardiac arrest following the injection of suxamenthonium in a severely burned patient has been reported by Allen *et al* (1961), Bush (1964) and Tolmie *et al* (1967). Both the bradycardia and arrhythmia associated with suxamethonium can be antagonized by the intravenous injection of atropine, and it is the author's practice to give this drug after an injection of suxamethonium if the heart rate falls to 40 beats per minute or if the rhythm becomes irregular. Atropine sulphate 0·65 mg. diluted to 4 ml. with N-saline should be available prior to induction of anaesthesia and 1 ml. doses should be injected intravenously when indicated.

It has been demonstrated that the administration of suxameth-onium to the fully digitalized patient can produce dangerous ventri-cular arrhythmias and that these arrhythmias can be abolished by the injection of d-tubocurarine. In the partially digitalized patient it produces changes characteristic of digitalization. It has also been shown that the arrhythmias of digitalis intoxication in dogs and cats can be abolished by d-tubocurarine and it has been suggested that digitalis, acetylcholine and suxamethonium may produce the same myocardial transmembrane ionic flux which is responsible for ventricular fibrillation (Dowdy and Fabian 1963).

Suxamethonium should be used with care in the patient who is receiving quinidine as this alkaloid has a depressant effect on skeletal as well as cardiac muscle. It acts both directly on the muscle fibre and on neuromuscular transmission at the motor end plate and prolonged apnoea may follow (Grogono 1963). Similar vigilance should be exercised when the non-depolarising relaxants are used in the patient receiving quinidine (Way and Larson 1967). Suxamethonium may be potentiated both by tacrine hydrochloride and hexafluorenium but cardiac arrhythmia has only been asso-ciated with the latter agent (Duncalf et al 1965).

INHALATIONAL AGENTS

The effect of these on the ECG varies. Some, like nitrous oxide in the presence of adequate oxygenation and ventilation produce no effects whereas others like chloroform and cyclopropane may pro-duce dangerous arrhythmias.

The changes are due to either vagal stimulation or sympathetic activity or a combination of both. Vagal stimulation results in a bradycardia with a reduction in the height of the P wave. If the stimulus is marked and unopposed partial or complete heart block or even asystole may occur. Sympathetic overactivity, on the other hand, results in a tachycardia, with an increase in the height of the P wave and occasional ventricular extrasystoles. If the stimulus is marked and unopposed the ventricular extrasystoles become more frequent and may develop into the multifocal variety which may be the precursor of ventricular fibrillation.

CHLOROFORM

Levy (1914) postulated ventricular fibrillation as the cause of sudden death during induction with chloroform, and the classical work of Hill (1932a, b) demonstrated multifocal ventricular tachycardia in about 50% of cases during induction and that the arrhythmia disappeared as anaesthesia was deepened.

The liberation of endogenous adrenaline from the suprarenal by fear, pain, hypoxia, CO_2 retention or the injection of adrenaline by the surgeon may act on a chloroform sensitized myocardium to precipitate a dangerous or even fatal ventricular arrhythmia.

Vagal stimulation may also be a cause of death (Waters 1951). During induction with chloroform a period of breath holding when using the open drop method of administration could result in the build up of an irritant concentration of vapour which when the patient starts breathing again could so stimulate the pulmocardiac reflex that asystole results. To reduce these hazards, chloroform should be administered through an accurately calibrated vaporiser, such as a Chlorotec, and the patient should be adequately premedicated, induced with an intravenous barbiturate, well oxygenated and ventilated. With all these precautions however, cardiac arrest can still occasionally occur (Hart and Duthie 1964) and in the author's view chloroform should be eliminated from modern anaesthetic practice.

ETHYL CHLORIDE

This agent should be treated with the same respect as chloroform for its administration carries similar risks and its use should now be restricted to the production of localised refrigeration analgesia.

TRICHLORETHYLENE

Almost every known form of cardiac arrhythmia has been reported during anaesthesia with this agent and Orth (1958) found ECG evidence of irregularities in about two-thirds of patients.

It is now however only used as an analgesic supplement and provided hypoxia and CO_2 retention do not occur and adrenaline is avoided (Matteo et al 1962) arrhythmias in these light levels of anaesthesia are rarely observed.

Should higher concentrations be inadvertently used tachypnoea and CO_2 retention occurs with the resultant appearance of ventricular arrhythmias but these can be abolished by the intravenous injection of pethidine (Johnstone 1951b).

DI-ETHYL-ETHER

From a practical point of view this agent is probably still the safest although the deliberate forced inflation of a high concentration of vapour may so stimulate the pulmocardiac reflex that asystole results. This is more likely to occur when the larynx has been paralysed by a relaxant.

Ether may cause an alteration in the height of the P wave, a wandering pace maker and occasional ventricular extrasystoles, but these are of no particular significance and may occur under any type of anaesthesia. Adrenaline in normal dosage may safely be used in the presence of this agent.

DIVINYL ETHER

This and methyl-N-propyl ether behave in a similar way to di-ethyl-ether and do not sensitise the myocardium to the effects of adrenaline.

A case of atrial flutter has however been reported but here the divinyl ether was given for a prolonged period in a closed circuit (Johnstone 1951a).

METHOXYFLURANE

This fluorinated ether, in its cardiovascular effects, resembles halothane rather than ether but does not sensitise the heart to adrenaline (Hudon 1961). No characteristic ECG changes have been reported in man.

HALOTHANE

Since its introduction in 1956 halothane has become the most widely used inhalational anaesthetic.

The vagal effects of this agent are common and if the heart rate falls to 40 beats per minute it should be corrected by the intravenous injection of 0.15 mg of atropine sulphate.

Sympathetic effects also occur. Ventricular extrasystoles are common if CO_2 retention is allowed (Black *et al* 1959; Fukushima *et al* 1968). Only rarely however have ventricular extrasystoles of the multifocal variety been seen (Payne and Plantevin 1962).

Occasionally intubation under halothane has produced a ventricular arrhythmia (Burnap *et al* 1958; Delaney 1958), while stretching of the anal sphincter may produce a similar effect (Gauthier *et al* 1962).

That the use of adrenaline in the presence of halothane could induce ventricular extrasystoles and ventricular tachycardia was demonstrated by Brindle *et al.* (1957). More recently three cases of cardiac arrest have occurred, two following reconstructive operations on the vagina (Rosen and Roe 1963), and one during the vaginal part of an abdomino-vaginal hysterectomy (de Lange 1963). The speed with which the arrests occurred suggests the accidental intravenous injection of adrenaline which is especially likely to occur in the erectile tissue of the external genitalia of both sexes, in the broad ligaments of the uterus, in the neck and suboccipital area. In the presence of halothane the injection of adrenaline should either be avoided (Davies 1965) or be restricted to the subcutaneous tissues and injected in a concentration not exceeding 1:100,000 at a rate not exceeding 1 ml per minute (0·01 mg) up to a maximum of 10 ml. in the adult under continuous ECG control (Katz *et al* 1962). The injection of adrenaline and CO_2 retention are, however, not the only causes of ventricular arrhythmias under halothane. Other causes include hypoxia, hypovolaemia, the intravenous use of atropine and sensory stimulation under light anaesthesia.

Much exodontia has been carried out under light halothane anaesthesia and gross ventricular arrhythmias have been observed in the cardiac patient (Kaufman 1966) and to a less severe degree in the normal patient (Forbes 1966).

As halothane both increases vagal tone and myocardial sensitation to catecholamines sympathetic stimulation from any cause

F

will facilitate the development of cardiac arrhythmia even in the presence of adequate oxygenation and ventilation.

It is, however, interesting to note that deep halothane anaesthesia has been used successfully for the surgical removal of a phaeochromocytoma without the appearance of any arrhythmia (Rollason 1964). Moreover it has been used for open cardiac surgery during which intracardiac adrenaline was used, but no ventricular tachycardia or fibrillation ensued (Orton and Morris, 1959; Dawson *et al* 1960). Nevertheless, the intrusion of frequent ventricular extrasystoles into the ECG pattern should be regarded by the anaesthetist as a warning signal not to be ignored and propranolol should be available (Johnstone 1966). In the unatropinized patient this drug should be given in small incremental doses of 0·25 mg. and atropine should be at hand to correct any bradycardia and hypotension.

Halothane in association with controlled ventilation can produce profound hypotension and this has been deliberately and successfully employed without any significant ECG changes for radical surgery in malignant disease of the face (Robinson 1964) but a very high alveolar oxygen tension is mandatory if cardiac arrest is to be avoided as cardiac output is very low.

Halothane facilitates the induction of moderate hypothermia and does not increase the incidence of ventricular arrhythmias provided the temperature does not fall below 28°C. (82·4°F.), good oxygenation and ventilation are ensured (Rollason and Latham 1963).

CYCLOPROPANE

This is the only gaseous agent which can produce serious cardiac arrhythmias.

Johnstone (1950) pointed out that ventricular arrhythmias are frequent during deep cyclopropane anaesthesia, but they can usually be prevented by adequate oxygenation. He also showed (Johnstone 1953) along with Matteo *et al* (1963) that these arrhythmias were frequent in the presence of intramuscular adrenaline and noradrenaline, but that that they could be inhibited by stimulating the pulmocardiac reflex with ether. Lurie *et al* (1958) have, however, shown that cyclopropane itself can produce ventricular arrhythmias in normal man not subjected to operation and in the presence of adequate oxygenation and CO_2 elimination. The presence of arrhythmia in these circumstances suggests a high cyclopropane concentration. Ventricular arrhythmias are common in the lighter levels of cyclopropane anaesthesia in the presence of CO_2 retention, and are further accentuated when an elevated pCO_2 is suddenly reduced and this is particularly so in the presence of the higher blood concentrations of cyclopropane. Price *et al* (1958), however, have found that bilateral stellate ganglion blockade with a local anaesthetic can render CO_2 retention relatively ineffective in producing these ventricular arrhythmias. In the patient under cyclopropane anaesthesia an injection of gallamine may precipitate a ventricular tachycardia and this relaxant should be avoided (Walts and Prescott 1965).

Intravenous atropine should also be avoided (Kristoffersen and Clausen 1967).

The incidence of cardiac arrhythmias during a straight cyclopropane anaesthetic is significantly higher than in a thiopentone-cyclopropane sequence, (Seuffert and Urbach 1967).

ADRENALINE AND NORADRENALINE

The use of adrenaline and noradrenaline can induce ventricular arrhythmias which may terminate in ventricular fibrillation during anaesthesia with chloroform, ethyl chloride, trichlorethylene, halothane and cyclopropane particularly if hypoxia or CO_2 retention is also present or if cocaine has been used topically. Some adrenalytic compounds such as perphenazine can suppress these adrenaline induced arrhythmias. Because perphenazine also has powerful anti-emetic properties it is the author's practice to use it both in premedication and in association with methadone in the early post-operative period. In the presence however, of a persistent ventricular arrhythmia propranolol should be used. This is most likely to occur in a patient with hyperthyroidism or with a phaeochromocytoma. In the latter instance, and in cases of accidental overdosage with adrenaline, phenoxybenzamine should be used in addition to propranolol (Glover and Shanks 1967).

ECG changes recorded during infusions of adrenaline and nor-adrenaline include depression of the ST segment, depression and inversion of the T wave and elevation of the U wave (Lepeschkin *et al* 1960).

It is possible that adrenaline and noradrenaline will be replaced by PLV-2 ('Octapressin') as this agent has been found to be a safe and effective local vasoconstrictor and its intravenous and sub-cutaneous injection during cyclopropane, trichlorethylene and halothane anaesthesia does not produce cardiac arrhythmias (Katz 1965; Lazar and Snider, 1966).

ANGIOTENSIN

This drug has been used for maintaining blood pressure after the removal of a phaeochromocytoma. Its use, however, may cause changes in the T wave and extrasystoles (Boek 1960).

SYNTOCINON

Pitocin has now been abandoned in obstetrics in favour of synto-cinon. The latter unlike pitocin has an antiarrhythmic action although its use may be associated with a slight fall in blood pres-sure and increase in heart rate (Katz 1964).

NEOSTIGMINE AND ATROPINE

These drugs continue to be routinely used to reverse the effect of curarization produced by non depolarising relaxants. Some inject the drugs together while others precede the administration of neo-stigmine by an injection of atropine. Usually no significant ECG changes are seen after either technique when the patient has been well oxygenated and ventilated (Rollason 1958; Riding and Robin-son 1961). In the presence of CO_2 retention, secondary to hypo-ventilation, ECG changes occur which involve most components of the ECG and include extrasystoles, heart block, gross voltage reduction and transient asystole. It would appear that in healthy patients the heart is protected from the effects of neostigmine by a respiratory alkalosis. This unlike respiratory acidosis, appears to produce no significant ECG changes (Rollason and Parkes 1957). CO_2 retention however in the presence of adequate oxygenation does not appear to produce ECG changes (Baraka 1968).

In the presence of cyclopropane dangerous arrhythmias may also occur (Jacobson *et al* 1954).

Johnstone (1951) showed that ventricular arrhythmias can appear within 30 seconds after the intravenous injection of atropine in patients under cyclopropane-ether anaesthesia with CO_2 retention. These arrhythmias took the form of a multifocal ventricular tachycardia and the view has been expressed by Pooler (1957) that atropine in association with CO_2 retention is the cause of the sudden deaths following the simultaneous intravenous injection of neostigmine and atropine. This view is further substantiated by the fact that sudden deaths have occurred after the injection of atropine alone, before neostigmine was administered, at the end of abdominal operations for obstructive conditions in patients with electrolyte imbalance, tachycardia and CO_2 retention.

Neostigmine alone in a dose up to 1 mg. may be given intravenously in cases of intractable supraventricular tachyeardia.

CARBON DIOXIDE

The inhalation of carbon dioxide in oxygen produces a respiratory acidosis which causes a delayed conduction within the myocardium resulting in prolongation of the PR, QRS and QT intervals (Altschule and Sulzbach 1947; McArdle 1959).

Periods of paroxysmal tachycardia and atrial extrasystoles may also be seen. It should, however, be remembered that the absence of hypoxia and other complicating factors distinguish the dangers of inhaling carbon dioxide in oxygen from carbon dioxide accumulation during anaesthesia, where in association with hypoxia, electrolyte imbalance, atropine, and adrenaline, it may predispose to ventricular fibrillation.

It should also be remembered that the sudden reduction of a high CO_2 tension may predispose to dangerous ventricular arrhythmias.

Both CO_2 inhalation and a noradrenaline drip have been used to increase cerebral blood flow and maintain a high systolic pressure during the operation of carotid endarterectomy but ventricular arrhythmias are frequent and there is no concrete evidence that the technique is justifiable.

ELECTROLYTE IMBALANCE

POTASSIUM

Hyperkalaemia

A high serum potassium may be found in patients with Addison's disease, uraemia, shock, anoxia, dehydration, severe burns, and in patients on low sodium diets. It may also be seen in those receiving massive blood transfusions and in those on a KCl drip, particularly in the presence of inadequate renal function. Hyperkalaemia is characterized initially by tall peaked T waves which may be higher than the QRS complex. These are illustrated in Fig. 65.

Hypokalaemia

A low serum potassium may be seen in patients with diabetic

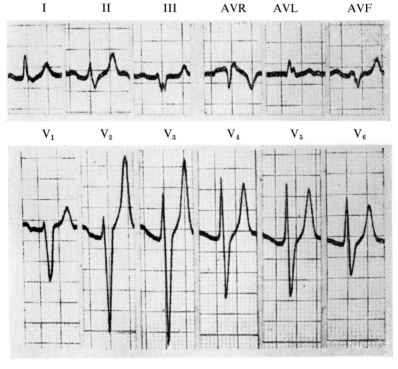

FIG. 65. Hyperkalaemia – serum K 7·6 m eq./litre – a case or uraemia.

acidosis, primary aldosteronism, potassium losing nephritis, excessive diarrhoea, and following the excessive use of steroids and certain diuretics. Hypokalaemia is characterized initially with prolongation of the QT interval, lowering or inversion of the T waves, and prominent U waves. These are illustrated in Fig. 66 and are best seen in lead V4.

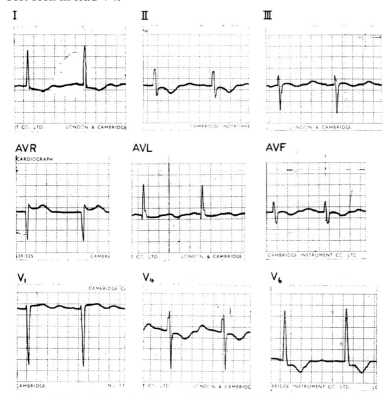

FIG. 66. Hypokalaemia—Serum K 1·7 m eq/litre—a case of chronic nephritis. Note depression of ST segments and T waves, prolonged QTc and prominent U waves especially in V4.

CALCIUM

HYPERCALCAEMIA

A high serum calcium may be associated with hyperparathyroidism. The QT interval varies inversely with the calcium level of the blood and in patients with a parathyroid tumour the QT interval

may be so shortened that the ST segment is abolished. This is
illustrated in Fig. 67.

HYPOCALCAEMIA

A low serum calcium may be found in hypoparathyroidism,
uraemia, after hyperventilation, vomiting and massive transfusion

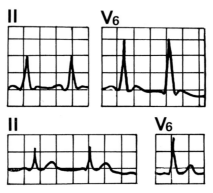

FIG.. 67 *Upper tracing:* Hypercalcaemia. Note absent ST segment and
short QT interval.
Lower tracing: Normal.

of citrated blood. The QT interval is prolonged but this is mainly
due to lengthening of the ST segment. This is illustrated diagrammatically in Fig. 68 where it is compared with the prolonged QT
interval associated with hypokalaemia.

CARDIAC DRUGS

DIGITALIS

This is the 'great imitator' and is to the ECG what syphilis has
been to medicine. Digitalis in therapeutic dosage most commonly
produces changes in the ST segment and the T wave. These changes
are as follows:

(1) Depression of the ST segment in those leads in which the
main deflection of the QRS is upright. The shape of the ST segment
is distinctive and appears as a straight line running obliquely
downward (the mirror image of a correction mark: ∨) or saucer-
shaped with the concavity upwards (Fig. 69).

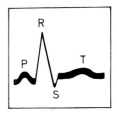 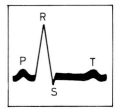

PROLONGED Q-T   PROLONGED Q-T

FIG. 68. *Left tracing:* Hypokalaemia (QT prolongation due to a low broad T wave).
Right tracing: Hypocalcaemia (QT prolongation due to a lengthened ST segment).

I   II   III   AVR   AVL   AVF

V₁   V₂   V₃   V₄   V₅   V₆

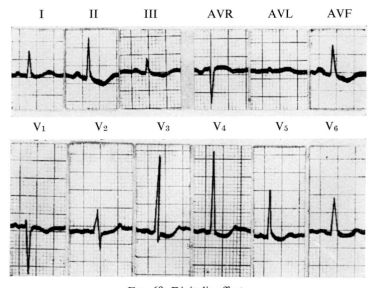

FIG. 69. Digitalis effect.

(2) Decrease in amplitude or even inversion of the T wave.

(3) Shortening of the QT interval.

Overdigitalization may produce various degrees of AV block, ventricular extrasystoles, often with coupled rhythm (pulsus bigeminus), nodal rhythm, atrial fibrillation, atrial tachycardia, ventricular tachycardia and, rarely, ventricular fibrillation.

Pulsus bigeminus is illustrated in Fig. 70.

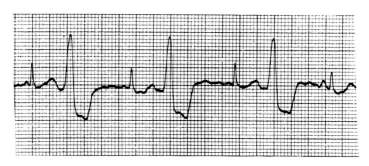

FIG. 70. Pulsus bigeminus.

<u>QUINIDINE</u>

ECG changes associated with therapeutic doses of quinidine are:
    (1) Prolongation of the QT interval.
    (2) Decrease in the amplitude or even inversion of the T wave, and
    (3) ST segment depression.

Excessive amounts of quinidine may produce various types of conduction disturbances, AV block, prolongation of the QRS interval, ventricular fibrillation or cardiac standstill.

Cases of paroxysmal ventricular fibrillation induced by digitalis or quinidine have been successfully treated with intravenous propranolol.

<u>PROCAINE AMIDE</u>

This drug should be administered intravenously at the rate of 100 mg. per minute in the adult under ECG control until either the arrhythmia for which it is being used is controlled or signs of drug toxicity such as ventricular extrasystoles, or a 50 per cent widening of the QRS complexes occur.

<u>LIGNOCAINE</u>

This drug has been widely used for the treatment of ventricular arrhythmias including those following bypass procedures (Weiss 1960). It should be administered in a dose of 1–2 mg. per kg. body weight at a rate not less than 1 mg. per minute in the same way as procaine amide and with the same precautions. Like procaine amide it may on occasion provoke ventricular tachycardia and fibrillation.

This drug is also used to produce intravenous regional analgesia in Bier's technique. Arrhythmias including a case of cardiac asystole have followed removal of the tourniquet (Kennedy *et al* 1965). Prilocaine appears to be devoid of these dangers.

The pain of angina decubitus has been successfully relieved by the thoracic epidural injection of carbonated lignocaine (Bromage 1967) and this resulted in an improvement in the ECG pattern. The attacks of pain were associated with a rapid thready pulse and flattened or inverted T waves but following epidural block of the first four thoracic segments the pulse slowed and the T waves returned to normal.

ISOPRENALINE

This drug increases the heart rate and stroke volume. It reduces peripheral vascular resistance, dilates the bronchial tree and does not cause potassium release from the liver. It is the drug of choice in the treatment of complete heart block occurring during open cardiac surgery and following myocardial infarction. As an emergency measure it should be infused intravenously (2 mg. in 500 ml. of 5 per cent dextrose) under ECG control while arrangements are made for pacemaking. When the latter cannot be done under fluoroscopic control successful placement of the electrode can be achieved by using the intracavitary ECG picked up by the pacemaker electrode as a guide (Bay and Sivertssen 1967).

Atropine, ephedrine and prednisolone may also be used in the treatment of complete heart block.

PROPRANOLOL

This beta blocker is a useful drug to control tachycardia and intractable ventricular arrhythmias including ventricular fibrillation. It should always be available and administered under ECG control.

In the presence of propranolol haemorrhage results in coronary vasoconstriction.

CHAPTER V

THE ECG DURING ANAESTHESIA AND SURGERY

Within the operating theatre the ECG differs in two important aspects from one recorded in the out-patient clinic or ward. The first of these is the greater opportunity for the introduction of artefacts, and the second is the rapidly changing pattern of the recorded signal due to the effects of anaesthesia and surgery.

During anaesthesia and surgery conditions are frequently changing; there are alterations in the concentration of the anaesthetic agents administered, manoeuvres such as intubation, alterations in posture, respiration, temperature, blood pressure and pulse rate. Monitoring the ECG is of importance in certain anaesthetic techniques, in certain major and minor surgical procedures, and in emergencies which may arise in the theatre. These will be considered in turn in this Chapter.

I. ECG CHANGES PECULIAR TO THE THEATRE SUITE

1. ARTEFACTS

AC INTERFERENCE OR 'HUM'

They may be produced by endoscopes *in situ*, e.g. bronchoscopes and cystoscopes when using mains reduction; by inadequate earthing of the ECG; or by inadequate earthing of other electrical apparatus, e.g. an electric blanket in use on the operating table. Interference produced by 50-cycle AC is illustrated in Fig. 61.

DIATHERMY CURRENT

The high frequency vibrations of the diathermy current completely obliterate the cardiac potentials and such interference is illustrated in Fig. 71.

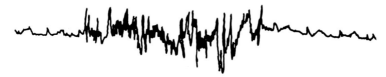

FIG. 71. Diathermy effect.

METAL OBJECTS

Large steel retractors, metal suckers and scissors in contact with the patient may induce static charges or may short circuit the cardiac potentials resulting in deflections which simulate extrasystoles (Fig. 72).

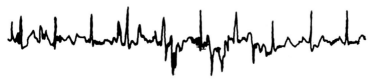

FIG. 72. Artefacts produced by retractors, metal suckers and scissors.

MUSCLE TREMOR

This may follow an injection of suxamethonium or be associated with shivering during the induction of hypothermia or during the subsequent rewarming. It may simulate fibrillary and ectopic atrial contractions which completely obscure the P waves, and is illustrated in Fig. 57.

DIAPHRAGMATIC CONTRACTIONS

These may be produced during a period of hiccoughs and during periods of tachypnoea associated with trichlorethylene or halothane anaesthesia and cause deflections which may resemble atrial ectopic beats (Fig. 73).

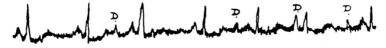

FIG. 73. Deflections produced by diaphragmatic contractions (D).

IDENTIFICATION OF ARTEFACT

There is no single technique by which artefact can be recognised and eliminated. Very low or very high voltage in the recorded signal and abnormal wave forms different from the patient's preoperative tracing should cause the anaesthetist to suspect artefact.

2. INTUBATION, ENDOTRACHEAL SUCTION AND EXTUBATION

In the author's view significant ECG changes during intubation, endotracheal suction and extubation are extremely rare in the absence of hypoxia, electrolyte imbalance, CO_2 retention or cardiac disease. When changes are observed, tachycardia, bradycardia, atrial, nodal and ventricular extrasystoles, atrial fibrillation, nodal rhythm, heart block, decrease in height of the T wave and depression of the ST segment are most common (Rollason and Hough, 1957a; Noble and Derrick 1959; Johnstone and Nisbet 1961; and Hutchinson 1967).

Cardiac arrest on rare occasions has been associated with these manoeuvres. In the severely burned patient the risk is greater (Fleming *et al* 1960; Bush *et al* 1962). The manoeuvres often produce a marked pressor response (King *et al* 1951; Rollason and Hough 1957a).

3. POSTURE AND CONTROLLED RESPIRATION

Changing the patient's posture, e.g. into the lateral or Trendelenburg positions may result in axis deviation. The employment of controlled respiration with deep inflation made possible by complete curarization or deep anaesthesia may also result in axis deviation and this is illustrated in Fig. 74.

II. ECG CHANGES ASSOCIATED WITH SPECIAL ANAESTHETIC TECHNIQUES

INDUCED HYPOTENSION

A comprehensive review of hypotensive anaesthesia by Larson (1964) suggests that this technique can be highly successful in skilled hands. Success is related to efficient continuous monitoring of the patient and the ECG plays a vital role in detecting arrhythmias and in some cases myocardial ischaemia. Change in the ST segment and the T wave provide evidence of possible myocardial

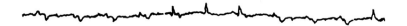

FIG. 74. Changes in electrical axis produced by controlled respiration.

ischaemia and call for immediate increase in the BP (Figs. 75 and 76). The ganglionic drugs *per se* do not appear to produce changes in the ECG.

It has been shown that ECG changes are significantly higher and their magnitude greater when the hypotension is associated with tachycardia (Rollason and Hough 1959, 1960a and b) Fig. 77. This suggests the use of agents such as halothane and techniques such as epidural and spinal which are associated with a bradycardia.

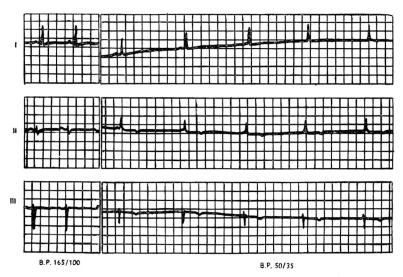

B.P. 165/100   B.P. 50/35

FIG. 75. Transitions from sinus to superior nodal, nodal and inferior nodal rhythm during the hypotensive phase. T wave flattening and inversion are also seen.

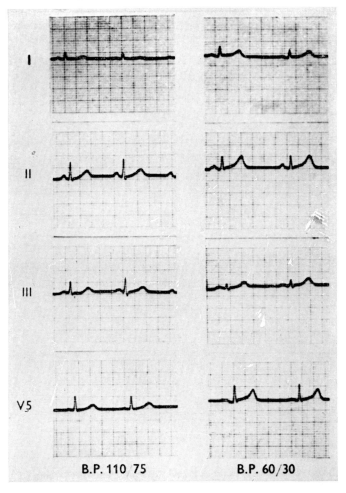

FIG. 76. Elevation of the ST segment and increase in the height of the T wave during the hypotensive phase.

The incidence of ST and T wave changes is greater when the rate of fall of BP is rapid (Rollason 1965). Figs. 78 and 79.

In order to corret the tachycardia sometimes associated with hypotensive anaesthesia propranolol may be used (Hewitt *et al.* 1967).

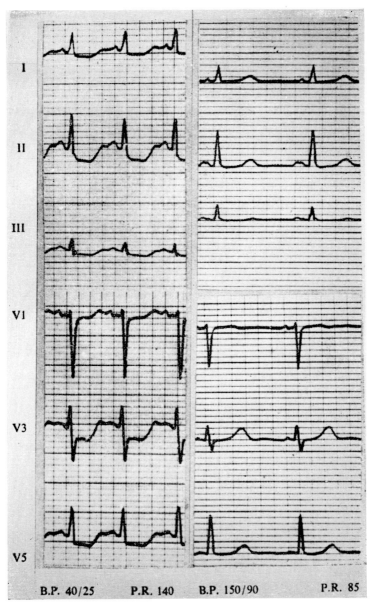

FIG. 77. *Tracings on the left:* Illustrate the gross ST depression which can be associated with a combination of tachycardia and hypotension.

Tracings on the right: Illustrate that these changes are reversible when the BP is raised and the PR slowed.

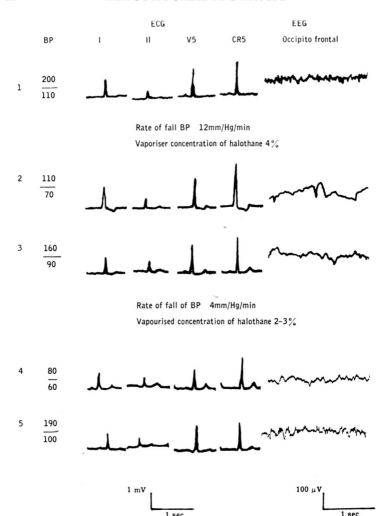

FIG. 78. In this 84-year-old man the BP initially falls rapidly (12 mmHg/min) and ST depression and delta rhythm become apparent. Halothane is then discontinued and the BP allowed to rise. This is subsequently lowered gradually (4 mmHg/min) but to a much lower level, yet the signs of ischaemia previously seen do not appear. It will be observed that the ECG changes are not apparent in lead II, the one commonly used by investigators, and stresses the importance of not relying on a single lead.

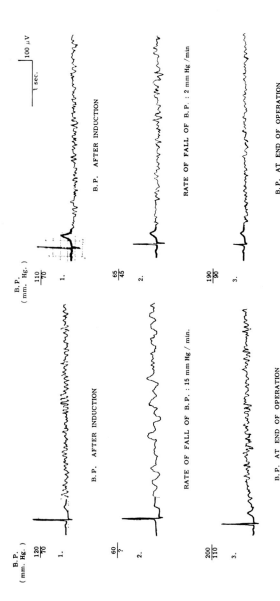

FIG. 79. This 80-year-old man was found at operation to have an oedematous retropubic space, apparently due to infection (tracing on left). Prostatectomy was accordingly postponed and sub-sequently carried out two months later (tracing on right). This patient thus acted as his own control. The ECG (lead II) and the EEG (occipito-frontal) tracings differ markedly on the two occasions. It is suggested that the ST segment depression and the delta rhythm noted on the first occasion were due to a too rapid fall in BP (15 mmHg/min) and the absence of changes on the second occasion, although the BP was reduced to virtually the same level, was due to the more gradual lowering of the BP (2 mmH/ming).

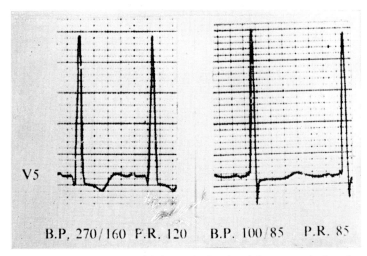

B.P. 270/160 P.R. 120   B.P. 100/85   P.R. 85

Fig. 80. Disappearance of left venticular 'strain' pattern during the
hypotensive phase in a case of malignant hypertension. The improved
pattern is probably due to a relatively greater reduction in cardiac
work than coronary flow. Slowing of the P.R. may also be a factor.

On occasions hypotensive anaesthesia may in fact improve the
ECG pattern in patients with gross hypertension (Fig. 80).

Profound hypotension has been used for radical surgery of the
face without ECG evidence of ischaemia (Robinson 1964).

INDUCED HYPOTHERMIA

Because of the danger of ventricular fibrillation it is essential to
continuously monitor the heart during hypothermia. ECG changes
usually commence with sinus bradycardia and reduction in the
height of the P wave but above 28°C ECG changes are not usually
significant. As the temperature drops the QRS interval gradually
lengthens followed by lengthening and depression of the ST segment and T wave changes (Fig. 81). At lower temperatures the
PQRST complex tends to become unrecognisable and arrhythmias
develop. These take the form of atrial fibrillation, extrasystoles, and
runs of ventricular tachycardia which end in ventricular fibrillation. It should, however, be stressed that ventricular fibrillation in
hypothermia can occur without any previous changes in the ECG

pattern. Fig. 82 shows a characteristic wave in the ECG tracing, the so-called J deflection first described by Osborn (1953) and seen during hypothermia. It was believed to be a current of injury, but now appears to have no special significance.

9·40
98·4°F M.H.

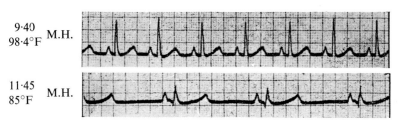

11·45
85°F M.H.

FIG. 81. *Upper tracing* is normal.
Lower tracing shows prolongation of the PR, QRS and ST intervals during induced hypothermia.

When hypothermia is used by itself, the customary limit of cooling is 28°C–30°C.

In profound hypothermia, the patient is cooled to 14°C and the ECG undergoes changes characteristic of cooling, bradycardia being followed by varying degrees of heart block, culminating in ventricular fibrillation or asystole. Atrial fibrillation is not as a rule observed. Occasionally the atria continue to beat at a slow rate in the presence of ventricular fibrillation.

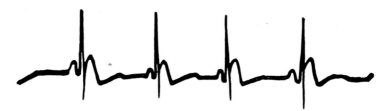

FIG. 82. The Osborn wave.

The ECG during ventricular fibrillation often shows a characteristic wave form of groups of complexes (Fig. 83). When this pattern has become well established, the ECG carries a good prognosis as defibrillation often occurs spontaneously on rewarming. During the period of circulatory arrest there is a state of suspended

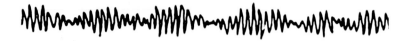

Fig. 83. Ventricular fibrillation pattern during profound hypothermia illustrating groups of complexes.

animation, cardiac and respiratory functions are in abeyance and the ECG unless the heart is fibrillating is isoelectric. Often fibrillation is not seen at any time during the operation, particularly in young children.

IIII. ECG CHANGES ASSOCIATED WITH SURGICAL PROCEDURES

CARDIAC SURGERY

Here the use of precordial leads is precluded and the anaesthetist must rely on the more remote limb leads. He has, however, the advantage of being able to observe the heart directly. Exposure of the surface of the heart to the drying action of the air and operating theatre lights, irritation of the myocardium by powdered asbestos, irrigating fluids, retraction, and the administration of drugs, such as digitalis, have all been observed to produce ST segment and T wave changes without any evidence of hypoxia or obvious alteration in the patient's clinical condition. The non-specific nature of these ST and T wave changes makes them a less reliable guide to myocardial oxygenation in the operating theatre than in the ward or consulting room. It is accordingly important to estimate myocardial oxygenation clinically by observing the colour of the heart and mucous membranes with a good light.

When, however, ST segment and T wave changes are associated with myocardial hypoxia, they are of the utmost importance and should be heeded without delay. If the hypoxia is due to respiratory obstruction or excessive hypotension, these must be remedied forthwith. If due to interference with the blood supply to a portion of the myocardium, as for example, during mitral valvotomy, when the descending coronary artery may be occluded by pressure, the surgeon must be requested to remove his finger or valvulotome for a while. On the other hand, the changes may be due to the clamp on the left atrial appendage involving the left coronary artery (Fig. 84(A) (B). If the ST and T changes appear just after the placement of an intracardiac suture, a coronary artery branch may have been occluded and the suture should be removed.

Different types of premature beat, atrial, nodal and ventricular are frequent during the surgical procedure, e.g. during cardiotomy in cases of atrial and ventricular septal defect, sub-valvular pulmonary stenosis and the Tetralogy of Fallot.

Should supraventricular tachycardia develop, and if the patient has received no previous digitalis, 0·5 mg. digoxin well diluted, can safely be given slowly by i.v. injection and repeated once if necessary after half an hour.

Short bouts of atrial fibrillation may also be observed.

When AV block develops the cause is usually apparent, for example, the placement of a suture in the heart may have interrupted impulse conduction within the bundle of His, or one of its branches. Removal of the offending suture usually results in the restoration of a normal conduction pattern.

Transient AV block or intraventricular block (idioventricular rhythm) frequently follows mitral valvotomy, but the normal conduction pattern returns soon after the surgeon's finger or vavlulotome is removed from the heart.

If complete heart block develops during an open heart procedure and does not respond to an isoprenaline drip, it may be necessary to treat it by suturing electrodes to the ventricular epicardium and connecting them to a pacemaker.

Ventricular fibrillation is not an infrequent accompaniment of cardiac surgery.

When hypothermia is used myocardial irritability is common. Cannard et al (1960) have observed that the heart is very irritable immediately following restoration of the circulation in operations for pulmonary valvotomy and in the repair of atrial septal defects (Fig. 85). All mechanical stimulation should be avoided following the release of the occluding clamps until the ECG shows less myocardial irritability as indicated by disappearance of the extra systoles and return to the control pattern.

Extracorporeal circulation is associated with ECG changes similar to those seen in other cardiac surgery. The stimulus produced by accidental compression of the great vessels or too prolonged handling often causes a sudden arrhythmia which disappears as soon as the stimulus is removed. The onset of supraventricular tachycardia with signs of myocardial failure call for immediate digitalization (Patrick *et al* 1957).

When direct coronary perfusion is employed, its adequacy can be determined by the ECG. The coronary perfusion rate is increased until the myocardium is pink and the ECG resembles the pre by-pass pattern. Should air inadvertently gain access into the coronary vessels, ischaemic changes will be observed.

In certain procedures, such as the correction of a VSD in children, some surgeons, in order to obtain a dry field clamp the

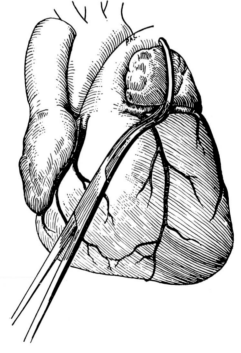

FIG. 84. (A) Clamp on the left atrial appendage involving the left coronary artery (B) ECG changes resulting from this.

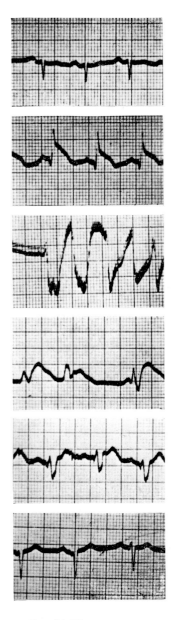

1. Tracing taken just prior to opening the thoracic cavity.

2. After occluding clamp applied. Note acute injury pattern simulating anterior myocardial infarction.

3. Ventricular fibrillation followed.

4. Position of occluding clamp was shifted and ventricular fibrillation ceased.

5. Temporary right B B B during closure of the atrial appendage.

6. During closure of the thoracic cavity the E C G returned essentially to normal and remained so.

Lead I taken in all tracings.

FIG. 84 (B).

aorta for periods up to 45 minutes. The ECG develops an ischaemic followed by a 'dying heart' pattern and may fibrillate or go into asystole, but quickly recovers normal sinus rhythm when the clamp is removed and the coronary circulation is restored (Fig. 86).

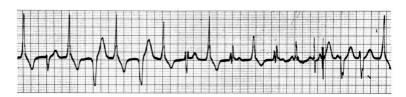

FIG. 85. Myocardial irritability immediately following restoration of the circulation.

During electrical defibrillation the ECG machine should be switched off to prevent damage to the instrument.

An unusual artefact has been reported by Cannard et al (1960) where a sine wave was produced by electrochemical potentials generated within the oxygenator (Fig. 87).

The operation for the insertion of a pacemaker for Stokes Adams disease should be performed under continuous ECG monitoring. When a pacemaker is in use the ECG pattern is complicated by the pacemaker pulses (Fig. 88).

Stokes Adams attacks may be triggered by intubation and intra-abdominal manipulation. The insertion of the intraventricular pacemaker electrode prior to surgery may be indicated. In these circumstances the common earthing of the pacemaker and the ECG machine is of major importance as ventricular fibrillation may be caused by minor electrical leaks (Noordijk et al 1961).

NEUROSURGERY

For posterior fossa procedures and those operations in the sitting position is it advisable to monitor the ECG continuously as a non-specific early warning system (Whitby 1963). The absence of ECG changes does not necessarily indicate an adequate circulation. Air embolism may produce arrhythmias and, if large, acute cardiac failure. Runs of ventricular extrasystoles and marked bradycardia with or without idioventricular rhythm are dangerous and the surgeon should be warned immediately. The ECG differentiates between a true bradycardia and alternating ventricular extrasystoles; in the absence of an ECG these may be difficult to distinguish owing to the difficulty of palpating the extrasystoles at the pulse.

In the treatment of congenital hydrocephalus by the establishment of a ventriculo-venous shunt the ECG provides a useful means of locating the tip of the catheter in the mid-atrium. The usual practice is to use the tip of the catheter as an electrode in place of the right arm electrode and to observe either leads I or II. The catheter electrode is either a metal stilette inserted within the catheter or alternatively the catheter is filled with 3 per cent saline. The ECG pattern is very sensitive to the exact position of the catheter tip in the heart and no difficulty is found in locating the desired position (Richards and Freeman 1964; Frazer and Galloon 1966). This is illustrated in Fig. 89.

The ECG can also prove useful in localising the position of the catheter for monitoring the central venous pressure (Phibbs 1966).

ECG changes simulating myocardial ischaemia may be seen in patients with cerebro-vascular accidents. There is some evidence that in a proportion of the cases no myocardial damage has occurred (Heron and Anderson 1965), and such ECG changes may, in fact, be an indication for surgery but the ECG should be continuously monitored during any surgery performed.

CAROTID ENDARTERECTOMY

In patients whose cerebral blood flow is critical, such as those who have recurrent 'little strokes' and multiple extracranial cerebral artery occlusions, cerebral perfusion using a femoro-carotid bypass with a flow of 4·0 to 4·9 ml/Kg/minute has proved advantageous (Foote 1967). Hypotensive and hypocalcaemic ECG changes may, however, occur during the priming of the extra-corporeal circuit and these emphasise the need for continuous ECG monitoring during the procedure, particularly as these changes

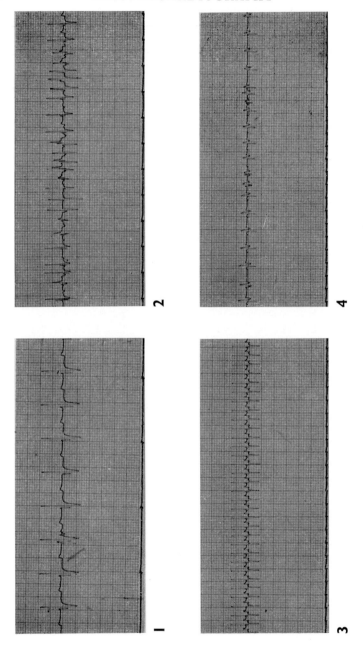

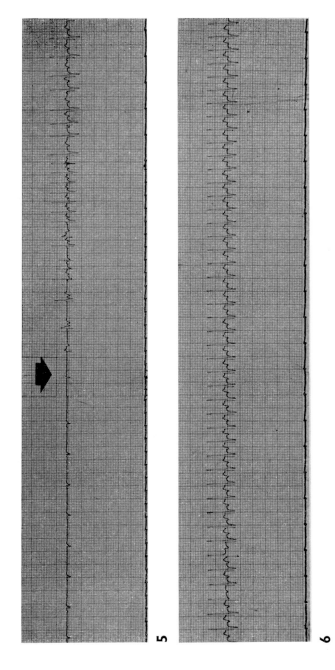

FIG. 86. ECG tracings during operation for closure of VSD and refashioning of pulmonary valve in a child. (1) Prior to application of aortic clamp; (2) shortly after application of clamp; (3) 2 min later; (4) 9 min after application of clamp; (5) to left of arrow: tracing when clamp had been *in situ* for 24 min; to right of arrow: tracing immediately after removal of clamp; (6) continuation of tracing (5).

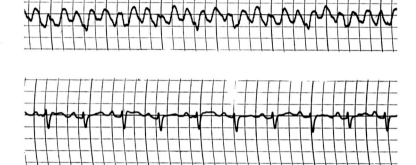

FIG. 87. *Upper tracing:* Sine wave artefact produced by pump oxygenator.
    Lower tracing: The true ECG picture.

can be rapidly reversed by the i.v. injection of 10 per cent calcium gluconate.

In less incapacitated patients, a simple shunt is used and during the endarterectomy cerebral vasodilation and systolic BP are maintained in some units by the combined use of CO_2 and a noradrenaline i.v. drip. In the presence of halothane, ventricular

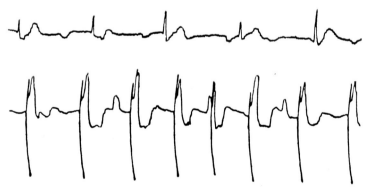

FIG. 88. *Upper tracing:* The true ECG picture.
Lower tracing: Artefact produced by an intraventricular stimulator (pacemaker).

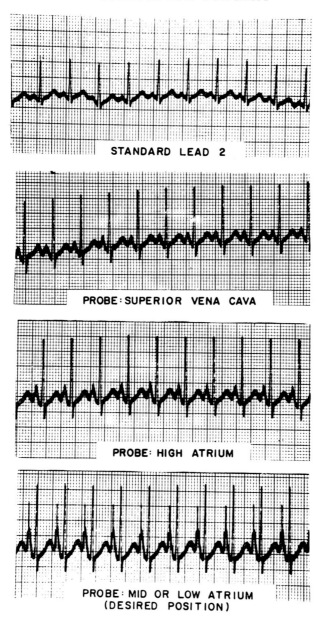

FIG. 89. ECG tracings illustrating intravascular recordings at various positions of the probe tip during catheter placement.

arrhythmias often develop, and emphasise the need for continuous ECG control.

Hyperkalaemia is always a risk with these patients and the ECG can be an effective means of monitoring this (Strunin 1966).

The use of stored blood with its high potassium content for transfusion may augment the risk and the appearance of tall tented T waves would indicate the need for the administration of calcium.

REMOVAL OF PHAEOCHROMOCYTOMA

The ECG should be continuously monitored during induction and maintenance of anaesthesia for this procedure. Ross et al (1967) enumerate the risks: hypertensive crisis after induction of anaesthesia (intubation), extreme fluctuation of blood pressure during the surgeon's handling of the tumour, arrhythmias from sudden release of large concentrations of sympathomimetic amines coupled with sensitization of the myocardium to production of arrhythmias by the anaesthetic agent, and sudden hypotension following removal of the tumour.

The cardiac arrhythmias are probably best left untreated unless they arise in the ventricles and are continuously showing the possibility of ventricular fibrillation. Extrasystoles and left bundle branch block may be associated with haemorrhage but tend to disappear with the rapid transfusion of blood.

OBSTETRICS

The study of the foetal ECG during labour provides one method of assessing the condition of the foetus. Parker (1965) has observed bradycardia associated with epidural block using lignocaine. Changes in the ST segment may indicate foetal distress as may extrasystoles (Smyth 1962).

Ebner et al (1960) studied the effect of post spinal hypotension on the foetal ECG and found that foetal bradycardia developed when the maternal systolic pressure dropped to 60 mm Hg for a period longer than 4 minutes.

EXCHANGE TRANSFUSIONS

The need for close acid-base control during exchange transfusion, coupled with the hazard of potassium and citrate intoxication, calls for ECG control during this procedure.

IV. MINOR PROCEDURES

CARDIAC CATHETERIZATION

During this procedure atrial and ventricular extrasystoles are common. If a dangerous arrhythmia, such as multifocal ventricular estrasystoles, develops the catheter should be immediately withdrawn until the tip lies outside the heart, and the patient should be ventilated with pure oxygen, even though the blood gases at that stage have not been estimated.

CORONARY ANGIOGRAPHY

This should also be conducted under continuous ECG control, particularly when hypotension is employed during the injection of the contrast medium. The systemic blood pressure can quickly be reduced by up to 50 per cent by inflation of the lungs with a constant pressure of 40 cm. water during suxamethonium apnoea (Malstrom et al 1960). When, however, abnormalities due to depressed conduction or ST deviation develop and are not obviously due to hypoxia which can be quickly remedied the investigation should be abandoned.

Some patients undergoing this procedure may have a high pulmonary vascular resistance and equally balanced left to right and right to left shunting, and under these circumstances the institution of controlled ventilation may result in a sudden fall of arterial oxygen saturation with bradycardia and ECG changes indicative of myocardial ischaemia.

CARDIOVERSION

This should be undertaken with a D.C. defibrillator with a built in synchronizer and cardioscope. (Fig. 94 (B).)

This is not usually carried out with ECG monitoring but cardiac asystole may occur during the clonic phase of the convulsion, when atropine has not been administered beforehand (Dobkin 1959) and it has been recommended that this drug should be given intravenously 75 seconds prior to the shock (Clement 1962).

When atropine is contraindicated intravenous lignocaine has been shown to be a satisfactory alternative. This drug reduces both the duration of the somatic convulsions and the incidence of arrhythmia. (Usubiaga et al 1967).

ECG monitoring in the post convulsive phase has revealed an increased incidence of atrial and ventricular arrhythmias after thiopentone as compared with methohexitone and that multifocal ventricular extrasystoles only occurred after thiopentone (Pitts et al 1965).

Following the rapid injection of propanidid, atropine and suxamethonium from the same syringe two in a series of 50 patients developed transient ECG changes. One with aortic valve disease had isolated ventricular extrasystoles and the other a supraventricular tachycardia and right bundle branch block (Jackson and Woodhead 1967).

V. EMERGENCIES IN THE OPERATING THEATRE

CARDIAC ARREST

The value of the ECG changes in cases of cardiac arrest is to ascertain whether the heart is in asystole or ventricular fibrillation and subsequently to assess the effectiveness of remedial measures such as thumping the precordium (Baderman and Robertson 1965), the correction of metabolic acidosis (Stewart et al 1965), the use of the pacemaker for asystole, and the DC defibrillator for ventricular fibrillation.

For the poor risk patient continuous ECG monitoring should reduce the hazard of cardiac arrest. Experience has shown that the following conditions may on occasion produce cardiac arrest:—

(1) Endotracheal intubation.

(2) Endoscopy, e.g. bronchoscopy; cystoscopy and sigmoidoscopy in paraplegics with lesions above D6.
(3) Ocular surgery due to the oculocardiac reflex (Pöntinen 1966).
(4) Denervation of a hypersensitive carotid sinus.

PULMONARY EMBOLISM

This produces a characteristic series of ECG changes which in addition to right heart 'strain' (Fig. 30) include a large P pulmonale in leads II and III, a prominent S wave in lead I, a deep Q wave and inverted T wave in lead III (Fig. 90).

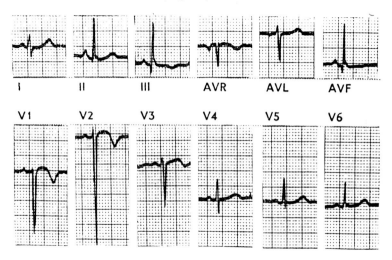

FIG. 90. Acute pulmonary embolism. Note S1, Q3, T3 pattern, right axis deviation and T wave inversion and raised ST segments in leads V1 and V2.

TRANSFUSION THERAPY

Some cases of cardiac arrest encountered during anaesthesia appear to be due to massive blood transfusion or to the transfusion of concentrated or fresh frozen plasma. The critical factor suggested is the ratio of potassium to calcium in the venous return to the heart. The anaesthetist when supervising one of these transfusions should have the benefit of continuous ECG control.

Should tall tented T waves and prolonged QT intervals develop during the transfusion of blood or plasma, particularly in small children whose reservoir of tissue in relation to their blood volume is small, it would appear advisable to inject ten per cent calcium gluconate or chloride slowly intravenously *pari passu* with the blood or plasma until the ECG changes are reversed. The development of gross ischaemic ECG changes should lead the anaesthetist to suspect air embolism.

The need for massive transfusion on the one hand must be weighed against the danger of circulatory overloading and pulmonary oedema on the other, particularly in chest injuries and during a pneumonectomy when the ECG should be observed for evidence of right heart 'strain'.

The massive transfusion of refrigerated blood may produce cardiac arrest (Boyan and Howland 1961) and a blood warmer should be used.

ECG changes may on occasion be associated with transfusions other than those of blood and plasma. Dehydration therapy with 30 per cent urea for instance may result in the appearance of elevated ST segments and inverted T waves.

CHAPTER VI

THE ECG AND INTENSIVE CARE

An intensive care unit should be ready to accept all patients needing the continuous support of a vital function or who are liable to do so at short notice. Conditions calling for intensive care include myocardial infarction, extensive burns, patients undergoing renal dialysis, and all conditions requiring artificial ventilation.

Although the need for such units has long been realised and some experiments have been made, it is only recently that such units have become routine in the larger hospitals. Thus it would be unwise to do more than suggest the utility of the ECG in these situations.

The prompt recognition of an arrhythmia and skilful treatment may well determine the success of the therapy.

Those patients whose condition on leaving the operating theatre gives ground for concern should be referred to the intensive care unit.

The ECG has proved useful in the following situations:

1. CARDIAC CONDITIONS

The continuous monitoring of the ECG here is obligatory and particularly in patients who have had a cardiac arrest, a coronary thrombosis or a cardioversion. It has been reported that in cardioversion the general anaesthetic produced no rhythm changes (Gilston *et al* 1965).

Aortic stenosis and ischaemic heart disease predispose to cardiac arrest.

2. RESPIRATORY CONDITIONS

In chest injuries, it has been pointed out (Campbell 1966) that serious cardiac injury is undoubtedly present more often than is generally realised. This means that the ECG should be certainly taken, but continuous monitoring will not be necessary in all cases.

In status asthmaticus it has been suggested that if isoprenaline aerosol by IPPR is administered, it is prudent to monitor the patient with an ECG during the administration and for at least ten minutes afterwards (Grant 1966). The same precaution should be taken if dilute adrenaline is given intravenously.

The onset of hypotension in patients with tetanus and polio-myelitis treated with IPPR may indicate the onset of myocarditis and suggests the need for ECG monitoring. On the other hand, some cases of severe tetanus may be associated with hypertension and ventricular arrhythmias which respond favourably to treatment with propranolol and bethanidine in addition to routine anticoagulant therapy (Crampton-Smith and Prys Roberts 1968). In the case of neonatal tetanus ECG abnormalities such as complete bundle branch block may be due to inadequate ventilation (Smythe 1963).

A technique combining both respiratory and ECG monitoring has been described (Farman and Juett 1967).

In the case of the respiratory distress syndrome of the new born ECG monitoring is desirable and it has been suggested that the ECG pattern can be used as a prognostic tool (Sutten and Heese 1964).

3. ELECTROLYTE IMBALANCE

Gross hypokalaemia can result in respiratory failure and may be due to such conditions as diabetes and potassium losing nephritis and replacement therapy should be carried out under continuous ECG control.

4. POISONING

In cases of severe barbiturate poisoning the patient may appear to be dead but the ECG tracing may be normal. Prompt treatment has led to successful recovery.

5. HYPERBARIC OXYGEN CHAMBER

When this is used for radiotherapy, anaesthesia is complicated because attendants are not allowed in the chamber. A system of remote control monitoring should include the ECG to monitor the action of the heart.

In carbon monoxide poisoning rapid improvement in the ECG pattern is a good prognostic sign.

When hyperbaric therapy is used for cyanotic infants prior to surgery or transposition of the great vessels monitoring the ECG by radiotelemetry has proved useful (Hill 1966).

In some patients a bundle branch block pattern has developed within minutes of entering the chamber and persisted throughout the period of treatment (Jones 1968).

COMPUTERS

Computing methods are now being applied to the ECG in the intensive care unit and these will enable prediction from signal analysis and the measurement of trends will provide earlier warning of impending complications, e.g. cardiac arrest (Bushman 1967; Cliffe 1967).

CHAPTER VII

THE ECG IN ANAESTHETIC RESEARCH

In research, the anaesthetist has two distinct aims:—firstly, the study of the physiological effects associated with both anaesthetic agents and drugs used in anaesthesia and, secondly, the improvement of anaesthetic techniques for the benefit of both patient and surgeon.

The ECG studies the electrical activity of the heart and there is no definite correlation between the ECG and heart function. Hence the first question to consider is what can be deduced from the electrocardiogram.

INFORMATION AVAILABLE FROM THE ECG

Typical patterns occurring in abnormal ECGs have been presented in Chapter III. During anaesthetic procedures the pre-existing ECG pattern may change and may simulate one of the abnormal ECG's. The interpretation of the changes needs caution, as marked ECG changes can occur without the corresponding physiological changes and, unfortunately, the reverse is also true. The following changes are likely to be seen during anaesthetic procedures:

(a) *Heart rate changes*

The ECG monitors heart rate efficiently and also gives an indication of the relative lengths of systole and diastole.

(b) *Onset of 'ECG myocardial ischaemia'*

The typical pattern of myocardial ischaemia may develop (Figs. 34 and 77). The electrical pattern is known to only occur for differential ischaemia namely, when the magnitude varies in different

parts of the myocardium; equally the pattern is not always correlated with other signs of myocardial ischaemia. However, in the
circumstances of anaesthesia, the onset of ST depression and T
wave inversion can reasonably be considered indications of in-
sufficient oxygenation of the heart.

(c) *Development of 'ECG cor pulmonale'*

This shows up as a pattern of right axis deviation, right ventricular
'strain', right bundle branch block, a prominent S wave in lead I
and a large Q and inverted T in lead III (fig. 90). This development
can usually be taken to suggest a pulmonary embolism. If this is
severe the pattern will change to that for cardiac arrest.

(d) *Ventricular fibrillation*

The pattern (Fig. 51) is quite clear and will quickly be confirmed by
other indications.

(e) *Ventricular standstill*

The absence of a QRS complex, even though P waves may be
present, means that the heart has gone into asystole.

(f) *Electrolyte Imbalance*

Figs. 65 to 68 show the characteristic changes associated with
electrolyte imbalance. The ECG can be a sensitive indicator of
these changes.

(g) *Development of heart 'strain' patterns*

This is associated with characteristic ST and T wave changes
(Figs. 29 and 30) and bundle branch block is often present as well.

(h) *Arrhythmias*

The main arrhythmias seen in the ECG are described on pages
35–52.

Unfortunately, many of those seem to have little significance under
anaesthetic conditions.

ANIMAL EXPERIMENTS

The ECG changes discussed above show that they cannot always be simply related to changes in the heart. The simplicity of ECG measurements makes them attractive and it is obviously useful to do experiments under conditions which permit their correlation with other measurements. In the patient, other interests exist beside research and hence it is valuable to do experiments on animals where the research can be carried through to its logical conclusions.

The use of animal experiment is two-fold: firstly, to persist in a technique producing ECG changes until serious consequences not detectable by other means manifest themselves. This shows that the ECG changes obtained are a useful warning and that it is indeed desirable to take steps to reverse them in clinical usage. In studying hypotensive anaesthesia, Rollason (1965) used the dog in order to be able to examine the ECG changes when hypotension caused myocardial ischaemia of such a magnitude that death ensued (Fig. 91(A) and (B)). Similarly Stewart *et al* (1965) wishing to examine extreme acidosis used bull calves.

Secondly, by using other measurements of heart parameters to see what actual heart changes, if any, correlate with the ECG changes (Fig. 92 (A) and (B)).

SPECIFIC ANAESTHETIC PROBLEMS WHERE THE ECG CAN BE USED

In all problems the ECG can be used in two ways:—firstly, to study possible risks to the heart, and secondly, to study methods of combating risks when they arise.

The main fields of research are illustrated below.

ANAESTHETIC AGENTS

One of the earliest ECG investigations during anaesthesia was that of Hill (1932a, b) on multi-focal ventricular tachycardia during chloroform anaesthesia. It has become normal to investigate the use of new anaesthetic agents by ECG studies; e.g. the examination of halothane by Johnstone and Nisbet (1961),

Not only have such studies shown the potential hazards of anaesthetic agents but they have been extended to demonstrate methods of either eliminating or treating them. The ECG is also useful for studying anaesthetic agents other than those producing general anaesthesia. For example, Kennedy *et al* (1965) and Kerr (1967) have used it in a study of intravenous regional analgesia using lignocaine and prilocaine.

DRUGS USED DURING ANAESTHESIA

The range of drugs used between initial premedication and the recovery room is extensive. All of them are administered for specific purposes and all of them may affect the heart, either in their own right or in association with the anaesthetic agent. Many investigations have been reported of drug activity, and it is not possible to review them all. Johnstone and Nisbet (1961) for example have shown the danger of adrenaline injections during halothane anaesthesia, and Dowdy and Fabian (1963) have shown that ventricular arrhythmias are produced by suxamethonium if given to a previously digitalised patient.

STIMULATION EFFECTS

The stimulation of the heart produced by endoscopy, oculocardiac reflex etc., causes ECG changes and so these may be used to study its magnitude and the efficiency of techniques designed to overcome the consequences. Jenkins (1966) has investigated arrhythmias during bronchoscopy and Pandit and Pandit (1965) have investigated the control of the oculocardiac reflex with gallamine.

Rollason and Hough (1957a) showed that many of the changes in the QRS complex seen during endotracheal intubation were in fact axis rotation and this shows the value of using a simultaneous 2-channel recorder in ECG research (Rollason and Hough, 1957b).

POSTURE

It has been suggested that postural changes may be dangerous during hypotensive anaesthesia and also that postural changes in

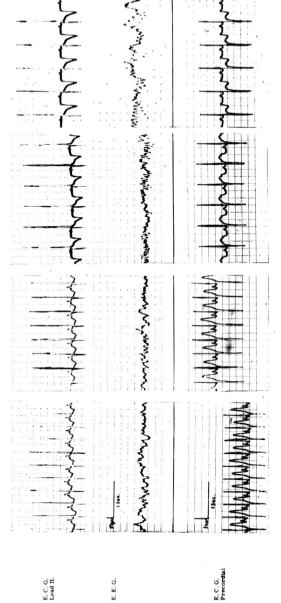

FIG. 91 (A) ECG changes illustrated in lead II and precordial lead and EEG changes (occipito-frontal lead) during increasing normovolaemic hypotension in a dog produced by halothane and IPPR. Other parameters simultaneously recorded include renal blood flow (electromagnetic technique), arterial and central venous pressure illustrated in fig. 92 (A) and (B). The six tracings were taken on a Devices 8-channel recorder (Fig. 96).

E. C. G.
Lead II.

E. E. G.

E. C. G.
Precordial

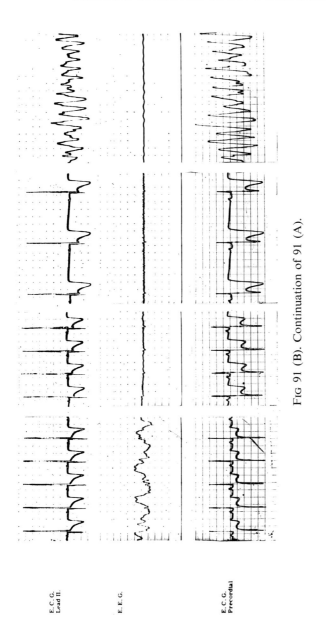

FIG 91 (B). Continuation of 91 (A).

E.C.G.
Lead II.

E.E.G.

E.C.G.
Precordial

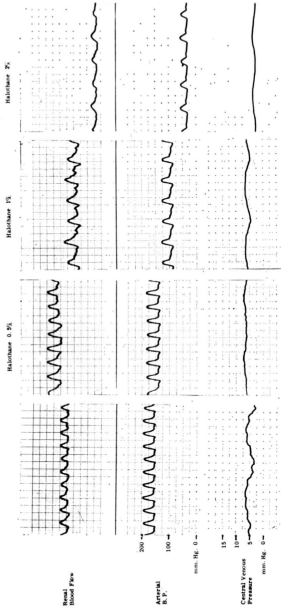

Fig. 92 (A)

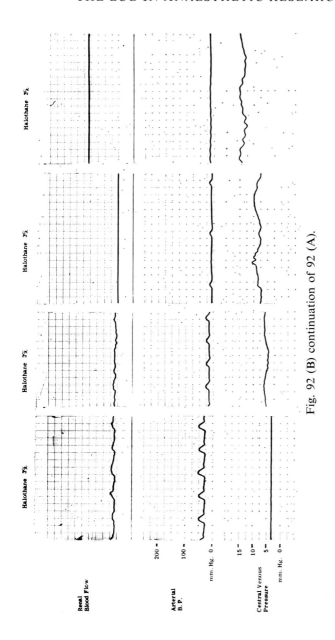

Fig. 92 (B) continuation of 92 (A).

the immediate post-operative period may be particularly hazardous. Whereas these changes may be more significant for the brain, the ECG offers a method of monitoring the heart during postural changes. Posture has been mentioned in the ECG literature but no major investigation seems to have been reported.

RESPIRATION

Under anaesthesia, carbon dioxide retention becomes a problem and so a major research topic in the study of respiration. Black *et al* (1959) used an ECG to study cardiac rhythm during halothane anaesthesia when hypercarbia was present; they found that atrioventricular nodal rhythm, ventricular extrasystoles and multi-focal ventricular tachycardia were associated with hypercarbia. Hence it is possible to check the efficiency of any ventilation system during halothane anaesthesia by examining the ECG.

HYPOTENSIVE ANAESTHESIA

Among the major risks of this technique is myocardial ischaemia if the hypotension becomes too great. The ECG provides one of the best simple monitors for this, and so has played a large part in research investigations on the safe use of hypotensive anaesthesia. One of the controversies about this technique is whether it is likely to increase or decrease the risk of anaesthesia in patients with a previous history of hypertension or coronary disease. The ECG has been used to investigate cardiac changes in such patients (Rollason *et al* 1964). Fig. 80 shows the improved ECG pattern observed in one patient.

HYPOTHERMIA

The ever-present risk of heart failure in hypothermia means that the ECG is a good research instrument. Development of cooling, and also of warming, techniques raises many questions which the ECG may be able to answer. Currie *et al* (1962) used the ECG to investigate the scope of surface cooling, using quinidine as a prophylactic agent against ventricular fibrillation. Rollason and

Latham (1963) used the ECG to investigate the safety of a combination of hypotensive anaesthesia with hypothermia for the treatment of intracranial aneurysms.

SPECIFIC SURGICAL TECHNIQUES

The dangers of cardiac arrhythmia during anaesthesia may, in certain cases, be more specific to the surgery than the anaesthetic procedure. The ECG can be used to investigate these risks:

Whitby (1963) for instance, has compared ECG changes during posterior fossa operations with other neurosurgical procedures. He showed that cardiac arrhythmias were likely to result when the surgeon was operating in the vicinity of the pons, the medulla and the roots of the 5th, 9th and 10th cranial nerves.

Again, Kaufman (1965) has shown that cardiac arrhythmia is liable to occur at the moment of extraction during dental surgery under general anaesthesia. An interesting feature of this report is that this original observation was made whilst doing routine ECG monitoring on bad-risk cardiac patients. Such arrhythmias, however, are less frequent during exodontia under general anaesthesia in the fit patient (Rollason and Dundas 1966, 1968)

CARDIAC ARREST

Clearly, the simplest indicator of both the onset of cardiac arrest and the success of therapy is the ECG. Many reports on this subject include ECG investigations; an interesting example is an account of a method of reviving the 'dead' by banging on the precordium. Baderman and Robertson (1965) illustrate the success of this technique by reference to ECGs.

ELECTROLYTE BALANCE

The ECG is one of the simplest methods of following changes in acid-base balance. Marshall (1962) has used the ECG to illustrate the ill-effects found in cases of massive blood transfusion due to excess potassium.

OBSTETRIC PROCEDURES

The effect of drugs administered to the mother by an anaesthetist on the foetus is clearly important. Parker (1965) has shown that

I

the foetal ECG may be used to study effects on the foetal heart. He showed that the administration of epidural lignocaine caused bradycardia in the foetus and that the intravenous injection of atropine to the mother reversed the effect.

These examples of the use of the ECG in anaesthetic research show that it is a useful tool, but that it has distinct limitations because it investigates the electrical rather than the mechanical efficiency of the heart.

CHAPTER VIII

ELECTROCARDIOGRAPHIC EQUIPMENT SUITABLE FOR USE BY THE ANAESTHETIST

It is difficult to make any recommendations for the type of equipment required by the anaesthetist as both the purpose and the resources in both money and personnel differ so widely. Valuable research has been done with the simplest equipment when the anaesthetist has had sufficient enthusiasm. It seems best, therefore, to discuss the ECG machines (electrocardiographs) in general and then to consider what features are particularly desirable for routine and research use.

ELECTROCARDIOGRAPHIC MACHINES

It is not proposed to give a detailed account of the design of ECG machines, as this would involve an unnecessary incursion into the field of electronics. An attempt will be made to describe the features which make certain types of machines particularly suitable for use by the anaesthetist.

The purpose of an ECG machine is to detect the changes of potential produced by the heart between two electrodes placed at suitable positions on the patient, and to make these changes visible to the observer. The potential to be detected is quite small, of the order of 1 mV, and the changes in potential occur rapidly (the QRS complex only lasts from 0·05 to 0·10 second) and is superimposed on the skin current which is DC potential. This may be as great as 20 mV, and varies slowly with time. The machine must separate the potential due to the heart from the skin current, amplify it, and then record the result (the electrocardiogram) in either a permanent or a temporary form. In the earliest types of

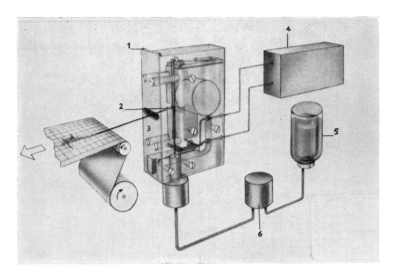

FIG. 93(A). The ink jet principle. (1) galvanometer casing (2) nozzle (3) jet of fluid (4) amplifier (5) writing fluid bottle (6) pump. A loop of wire is suspended in a magnetic field. Attached to this wire is a fine bore glass nozzle (2), weighing only a fraction of a milligram. When electric current is fed into the loop, it rotates, taking with it the nozzle. Writing fluid is supplied through a central capillary and during registration forced through the nozzle under high pressure (approximately 25 atmospheres) on the passing graph paper. The jet of fluid is only 0·01 mm in diameter and replaces the stylus arm used in conventional direct recorders.

machine, amplification was avoided by using an exceptionally sensitive detector—usually a string galvanometer.

All modern machines use an amplifier so that a less sensitive but more robust detector may be used.

The design of the electronic circuit will not be discussed, but the advent of transistors means that the circuit can be made both small and low in power consumption. The power is either from the AC mains or from a battery.

It is the recorder which is the aspect of greatest significance to the anaesthetist. If it is to follow faithfully the shape of the potential between the electrodes, it must be capable of travelling several centimetres in 0·01 second and be capable of making rapid

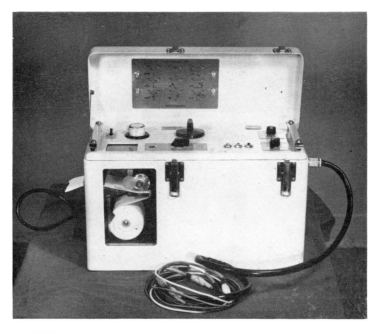

FIG. 93(B). The Mingograf 12 which incorporates the ink jet principle.

changes in direction without lag. Mathematicians have shown that it is possible to estimate the way in which a recorder will follow a complicated voltage pattern from the way in which it responds to simple sine waves of different frequencies. To follow the potential wave from the heart, the recorder should have a flat response from about 0·5 c/s up to about 500 c/s.

In a practical recorder this requirement has also to be related to the ease with which the recorder can be read. Four main types of recorder can be distinguished: (1) photographic, (2) stylus, (3) jet, and (4) cathode ray oscillograph.

The earliest type of recorder was the photographic. It has the great advantage that moving parts are light in weight and that the distance they move is magnified by the light beam; consequently it is not difficult to produce a recorder which has the required frequency response. The big disadvantage of this type of recorder is that the record is not immediately available and that a dark room is needed to develop the record. It is now possible to produce a special type of photographic recorder using ultra violet light and to make the record immediately available; such a recorder is more complex than the normal type and also more expensive.

The most common type of 'direct writer' ECG machine employs a stylus recording directly on paper. As the pen has to move several centimetres over paper during the recording of the QRS complex, it is difficult to preserve the finer details of the ECG. Most recorders of this type only record up to frequencies of 60–70 c/s. The stylus can be made to write by several methods but the most commonly employed for ECGs is a heated stylus writing on specially prepared paper. If an ink system is used difficulty is experienced in obtaining a uniform flow and also the frequency response of the recorder deteriorates.

An ingenious method of overcoming the poor high frequency response of the stylus direct writer is the use of a jet of ink in place of the conventional stylus (Figs. 93 (A) and (B)). The main difficulty with this design is that the galvanometer unit is liable to trouble with the jet becoming blocked, or if the ink reservoir is allowed to get too low.

Another method of recording ECGs is only a transient one, as they are displayed on the screen of a cathode ray oscilloscope with long afterglow. This makes it possible to see the ECG, but it soon fades away; it is usual to use this method to follow the behaviour of the heart over a long period and hence it has the name of 'monitor'. The great advantages of this method are that the picture on the screen is easier to see and no expensive paper is needed to record; during an operation of several hours duration, it would need several hundred metres of paper to keep a continuous record, and this is difficult to study as well as expensive. The 'Visicard 7' cardioscope (Kronschwitz 1964) by presenting a tracing direct from the thorax could prove time saving in emergency situations.

The availability now of using magnetic recording of the ECG signal as an intermediate store opens up interesting research possibilities. A lengthy procedure can be monitored visually and also recorded magnetically. Any interesting ECG changes observed can subsequently be selected from the magnetic recording and a permanent tracing made in the usual way. Ashton (1965) has described a complete system which also permits a rapid assessment of ECG recordings taken over a long interval.

All recorders are made in either single channel type or a type to record two or more ECGs simultaneously (multi-channel). Most of the multi-channel types can be adjusted to permit the recording of the output of other physiological parameters simultaneously with the ECG, e.g. the EEG and pressure measurements. It is of great value to be able to record simultaneously, as it permits the accurate correlation of the different parameters.

ECG MACHINES FOR USE DURING ROUTINE ANAESTHESIA

The value of having ECG monitoring available for major surgery is being realised; hence simple ECG monitors are becoming standard items of theatre equipment. It is not necessary to record ECG's unless they are required for research purposes, and so a direct writer is not an essential item of threatre equipment. As a major use of the ECG is in cases of cardiac arrest, it is very convenient to mount the ECG monitor in a resuscitator unit with the defibrillator, pacemaker, etc. (Figs. 94(A) and (B)).

In modern theatre suites, all the patient monitoring equipment is being removed from the theatres to a central monitoring room and a single display unit in each theatre monitors the physiological activity of the patient. This has great advantages in terms of both sterility and space saving in the theatres. Special cabling has to be provided between each theatre and the central monitoring room. The ECG is easily accommodated in this system and such a complex assembly will always be undertaken under the control of a specialist, usually the hospital physicist. To the anaesthetist, a centralised system will mean a lessening of the problems of ECG monitoring.

For some years to come it will still be necessary in many theatres to improvise, as neither of these systems will be available. A monitor is usually easier to accommodate if it does not have a stand. If no monitor is available, a direct writer ECG machine can

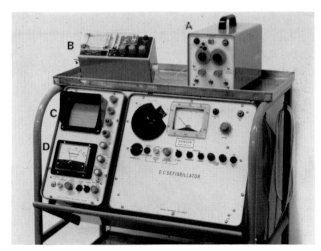

FIG. 94. (A) ECG mounted in a Resuscitator unit. A, Pacemaker;
B, ECG—direct writer; C, ECG—oscilloscope; D, heart rate meter.

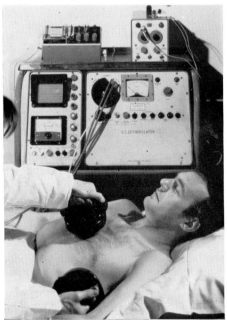

(B) ECG used in association with d.c. defibrillator to treat ventricular fibrillation.

be useful. ECG's are taken at intervals throughout the procedure and especially when it is thought possible that serious changes will occur. The use of ECG machines under these circumstances will call for the fullest co-operation of the theatre sister; this is most likely to be obtained through previous consultation.

ECG MACHINES IN THE INTENSIVE CARE UNIT

The ECG conditions in an intensive care unit are in general similar to those encountered by the cardiologist in his normal work. However, the long periods for which ECG monitoring is required means that monitors are more appropriate than direct writers; in order to keep a permanent record, ECG tracings will be taken from time to time, but the monitor is needed continuously. Most monitors provide facilities for taking ECG tracings with a standard machine. Some monitors are fitted with alarm signals which operate if the heart rate falls outside a predetermined range (Fig. 95).

In intensive care units, to reduce the need for staff, it is becoming a common practice to arrange that the physiological data for a group of patients is brought to a central monitoring point.

ECG MACHINES FOR ANAESTHETIC RESEARCH

For research purposes, it is not usually necessary to analyse the record immediately, so that the major disadvantage of photographic recording disappears and the very good record produced by this means is a real advantage. In research investigations, it is usually desirable to use a multi-channel recorder. Other variables of interest are EEG, arterial and central venous pressures, respiratory volume etc. It is standard practice to combine many of the instruments for recording these parameters into a single trolley. Most of these trolleys incorporate one or more oscilloscopes, so that it is possible to monitor variables and to record when there is an indication that significant changes are occurring.

The use of a single trolley with the complete physiological recording equipment on it has the great advantage that it simplifies the setting up of equipment in the theatre and also reduces the floor area required. Research is always an activity which tends to

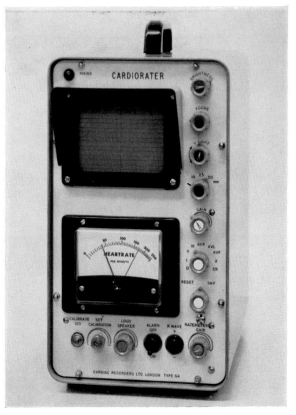

FIG. 95. Monitor fitted with alarm signals set to operate if heart rate falls below 40 or rises above 170/min.

conflict with the most efficient performance of routine surgery and all steps which reduce the conflict will assist in obtaining the willing co-operation of the surgical team which is essential if good research is to be done. A single trolley makes it easier for the anaesthetist to undertake the recording himself and certainly makes it possible to only need a single research assistant. Fig. 96 shows a typical trolley of a commercially available kind.

The analysis of ECG's taken during research investigations is a formidable task. Modern computer technology is very suitable for performing such analysis and the feeding of research physiological data directly to a computer or via a magnetic recording is coming into use. Mable (1966) has reported a method of transmitting ECGs via the telephone.

A most essential aspect of any investigation is to ensure that the equipment is in good working order and has been carefully set up and standardised before the start of the operation. It is never easy to arrange to make an adequate number of observations and it is very disappointing when observations during a particular operation have to be abandoned due to the failure of the instrument, or the results discarded because it is clear that the instrument was not correctly standardized. The most satisfactory procedure is to have the same team on all occasions and to work with the same theatre staff and surgeon; adequate time must be allowed for both the preliminary check of the equipment and also for setting up the final calibration in the theatre. It may well take five or six occasions

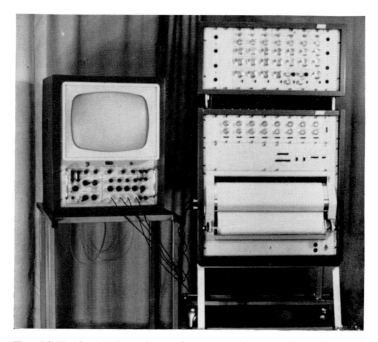

FIG. 96. Devices 8-channel recorder mounted on a single trolley and connected to an Airmec 4-channel oscilloscope.

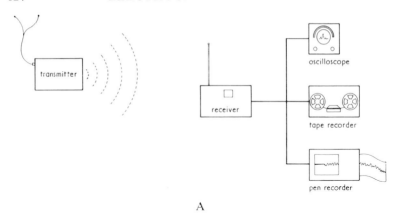

A

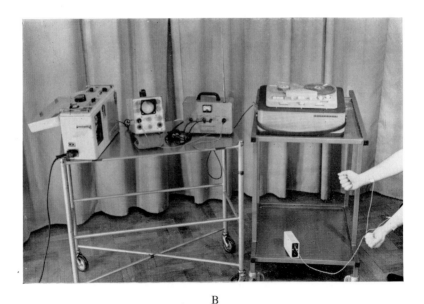

B

Fig. 97. Radiotelemetry system (A) Diagrammatic illustration of the system. (B) System currently used. From right to left: electrodes from patient connected to transmitter (in practice strapped to the side of the dental chair), tape recorder, receiver, Videoscope and Mingograph direct writer. (C) Tracings produced by the system compared with that produced by a conventional direct writer (top tracing).

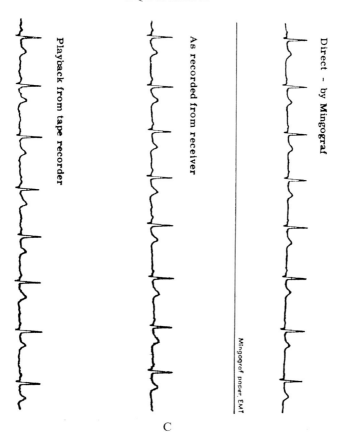

C

before the drill has been really well established and it will then be found that reproducible results can be obtained.

RADIOTELEMETRY

The miniaturisation of electronic equipment means that it is now possible to produce a transmitter weighing only an ounce or so to attach to the patient. The radio signal produced can then be picked up on a receiver and converted into the usual ECG displays. These systems have been widely employed for recording ECGs during normal activity and can have some utility in both anaesthetic and intensive care applications. They have been successfully used during dental anaesthesia (Fig. 97 (A), (B) and (C)) where patient movement makes normal ECGs difficult to record (Rollason and Dundas 1966; 1968). Radio waves will not penetrate steel and difficulty may be encountered if used between different rooms. The radio signal must be very weak or else a licence will be required as the signal will be picked up by other users of radio waves. The British Post Office has now allocated the band 102·2 to 102·4 mc/s for medical telemetry purposes.

ELECTRIC INTERFERENCE

ECGs are always liable to be marred by unwanted signals reaching the recorder. The design of the equipment virtually eliminates the DC skin potentials, but signals in the frequency range of the instrument will also be amplified and cause interference. Steps are taken in its design to reduce the unwanted amplification of the AC mains (common mode interference), but it will frequently be present in the tracing. The only further steps possible to reduce it are:

(1) To ensure good contacts throughout the circuit. The most likely place for trouble here is at the actual electrodes, but contacts between electrodes and lead, and lead and input terminal of ECG machines are also possible sources of trouble. A very difficult cause to detect is a partial break inside the lead; electrical stability has to be sacrificed to flexibility and so leads are liable to internal damage not detectable by the eye.

(2) Screening of the leads to prevent electrical pick-up along the length of the lead. An outer earthed conductor surrounds the active lead. In order to improve screening further a guard electrode system can be used. This uses a guard electrode situated somewhere on the patient connected to an extra screen inside the actual earthed screen. Just as poor contacts may occur inside leads due to invisible damage, the same effect may be found at the screen.

(3) Earthing connections must be very good or else these may also be sources of interference. The earth points of different equipment should go to a common earth point.

(4) Interference may be due to proximity of other sources of AC to either patient or leads. In the operating theatre comparatively little can be done about this type of interference but it is sometimes possible to re-route leads.

The reduction of AC interference is as much an art as a science; experience is the only method of dealing adequately with it.

In the theatre, there is that gross source of interference—the diathermy. When the diathermy machine is working, the ECG pattern either disappears completely or suffers from gross interference (Fig. 71). There is virtually nothing that can be done to eliminate this interference. The potentials induced can become so great that damage may be done to some types of machine. It is, however, possible to arrange a circuit such that when diathermy is in use it automatically cuts out the ECG machine.

ELECTRODES FOR ELECTROCARDIOGRAPHY

If interference is to be minimised good contacts to the patient should be made at the electrodes. The electrode resistance should be of the order of 2000 ohms and for anaesthetic purposes requires to remain in place for periods of several hours. The traditional electrodes for use in cardiological departments are very unsuitable for this purpose. Four types seem satisfactory for the anaesthetist.

(1) *The needle type*. This uses an ordinary hypodermic needle and is inserted into the skin. It is only suitable for use under anaesthesia but gives very satisfactory contact.

(2) *The disc (or button) type*. This comprises a stainless steel disc coated with electrode jelly and attached to the patient with strapping. Good contact can be made for periods of several hours.

(3) *The disposable electrode*. This is essentially a modified version of the last designed for use only once. An example of this type of electrode is described by Fluck and Burgess (1966).

(4) *The multi-point electrode of Lewes* (1965) eliminates the need for electrode jelly. Contact is made by using a large number of parallel point contacts most of which will penetrate the stratum corneum and hence reduce the skin resistance.

During surgery it is usually impossible to adjust electrodes and so great care must be taken to ensure correct application before the operation. The normal position of the limb leads may have to be varied, but provided they are attached to the limb or the trunk adjacent to the limb little error will be caused. The use of the right leg instead of the left will produce negligible changes.

It may sometimes be convenient during surgery to take an oesophageal ECG. A suitable electrode for this has been described by Kavan and Colvin (1965) and Inkster (1966).

An ingenious combination of a precordial electrode with a stethoscope has been described by Bethune (1965).

Occasionally it may be necessary to have a lead and its electrode sterilized and placed *in situ* by the surgeon.

In order to ensure the accurate placement of chest electrodes in the taking of serial ECG tracings, a grid has been evolved by Kerwin *et al* (1960) and a calliper by Rose (1961).

CHAPTER IX

THE VALUE AND LIMITATIONS OF THE ECG

The ECG provides the anaesthetist with a record of the heart rate, its rhythm, the site and number of the pacemakers, the efficiency of the conducting tissue and the position of the heart. It provides a means of recording fluctuations of autonomic tone produced by the various drugs used by him or his surgical and cardiological colleagues, and is a valuable index of the electrolyte balance of the blood. It is essentially a picture of the site of origin of the stimulus potential and the speed and direction in which it travels to initiate the myocardial contraction. As the conducting system and the myocardium derive their nutrient from a common blood supply, i.e. the coronary arteries, it seems reasonable to assume that any drugs or manoeuvres which produce electrocardiographic evidence of impairment of one may involve impairment of the other (Johnstone 1956). The ECG can be a valuable aid to the anaesthetist pre-operatively, during surgery and anaesthesia and in the post-operative period. The ECG changes, however, must be interpreted in the pre-operative period in conjunction with the clinical findings, in the threatre in conjunction with the events immediately preceding them, and in the post-operative period with the operation performed.

PRE-OPERATIVELY

The ECG can elucidate the following conditions:
1. Atrial and ventricular hypertrophy
2. Systemic diseases affecting the myocardium e.g. acute rheumatic fever.
3. Myocardial infarction
4. Pericarditis

5. Arrhythmias and conduction defects
6. Electrolyte imbalance
7. Effects of cardiac drugs
8. Coronary insufficiency and biliary disease.

DURING ANAESTHESIA AND SURGERY

Here the ECG is valuable:
1. In the evaluation of new agents, drugs and techniques.
2. In the detection of cardiac arrest and whether this is due to ventricular fibrillation or asystole. A case of cardiac arrest during anaesthesia and surgery and its response to cardiac massage is illustrated in Fig. 98.
3. As a continuous monitor during:
    a. Cardiac and vascular surgery
    b. Removal of a phaeochromocytoma
    c. Hypotensive anaesthesia
    d. Hypothermia
    e. Any type of surgery in the poor risk patient.

The development of the following should be viewed with concern and immediate remedial action taken:
1. Tachycardia above 160 beats per minute
2. Bradycardia below 40 beats per minute
3. Pulsus bigeminus
4. Multifocal ventricular extrasystoles
5. Gross ST segment and/or T wave changes and/or inverted U waves
6. Tall tented T waves with a prolonged QT interval
7. 'Dying heart' pattern or bundle branch block

The appearance of a right or left ventricular 'strain' pattern may constitute an indication for intravenous digitalization.

POST-OPERATIVELY

The prompt recognition of an arrhythmia and its skilful treatment may well determine the success of the surgical procedure (Buckley and Jackson 1961).

Drugs used to treat an abnormal rhythm should be administered not only under continuous ECG control but under the advice and guidance of a cardiologist. The treatment of fast arrhythmias may

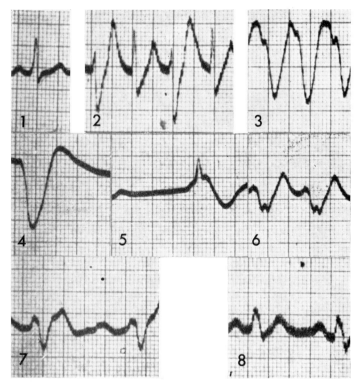

FIG. 98. A case of cardiac arrest occurring during anaesthesia and surgery. Lead II taken in all tracings. 1. Normal ECG 2. Multifocal ventricular extrasystoles 3. ventricular fibrillation 4. Massage contraction 5. Complex initiated by the heart 6. intraventricular conduction defect 7. conduction defect less marked 8. ECG at the end of the operation.

necessitate the use of such drugs as digitalis, quinidine, procaine amide, lignocaine and propranolol while neostigmine may occasionally be required. When arrhythmias are slow, as in various forms of heart block isoprenaline, atropine, ephedrine, adrenaline and prednisolone may be employed.

Electrolyte imbalance and metabolic acidosis may play an important part in maintaining an arrhythmia in which case such drugs as potassium chloride and sodium bicarbonate may help in its control.

K*

Atrial, nodal and ventricular extrasystoles which are initiated during a cardiotomy may persist for a day or two into the postoperative period.

The ECG should be checked twenty-four hours post-operatively in patients over 50 years of age with known coronary heart disease, hypertension, diabetes mellitus, peripheral vascular disease or abnormal pre-operative ECGs (Driscoll *et al* 1960).

LIMITATIONS OF THE ECG

The ECG only portrays the electrical activity of the heart and provides no indication of the strength of myocardial contraction and no record of haemodynamic events. Indeed, it has on occasion been known to provide a relatively normal tracing, certainly in a single standard lead, when the heart has ceased to beat effectively as a pump. An illustration of this is shown in Fig. 99. The patient had been clinically dead for some minutes when the relatively normal tracing was recorded and it was not until the lapse of a further half minute that this tracing changed into one of ventricular fibrillation. This hazard has been emphasised by other investigators (Mazzia *et al* 1966).

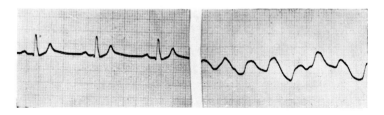

FIG. 99. *Tracings on the left:* Normal ECG tracing but patient clinically dead.

Tracings on the right: Taken 30 seconds later — ventricular fibrillation.

(Lead II)

On the other hand, the ECG may, on occasion, show grossly bizarre patterns in the presence of an adequate blood pressure. This does not call for panic, but the anaesthetist should ascertain the cause of the abnormal pattern and if possible remove it.

Finally, it should be stressed that the ECG should be used only as an ancillary aid and the anaesthetist should realize that it is no substitute for keen and constant clinical observation before, during and after surgery. The colour, BP, pulse rate, capillary refill time and pupil size should be frequently checked and take priority over any ECG tracings, except during periods of elective cardiac arrest.

APPENDIX

ARRHYTHMIAS OCCURRING DURING ANAESTHESIA

Type	Causes	Treatment
Extrasystoles		
(a) Atrial	Anoxia	Remove offending
(b) Nodal	CO_2 retention	stimulus
(c) Ventricular	Anaesthetic agents	Ensure adequate oxygen-
	especially chloroform	ation and CO_2 elimina-
	in the presence of	tion
	adrenaline	Correct electrolyte
	Atropine	imbalance and
	Digitalis	metabolic acidosis
	Metabolic derangement	Raise BP and tempera-
	Hypothermia	ture if indicated
	Intubation	Drugs: procaine amide
	Cardiac catheterization	quinidine
	Coronary angiography	lignocaine
	Cardiac surgery	propranolol
		Terminate surgery
Tachycardia		
(a) Supraventricular	Anoxia	Remove offending
(b) Ventricular	Haemorrhage	stimulus
	Drugs: adrenaline	Restore depleted blood
	chlorpromazine	volume
	gallamine	Carotid sinus and eyeball
	atropine	pressure
	Catheter in the heart	Drugs: vasopressors
	Surgical manipulation	digitalis (if not due to
	of the heart	digitalis toxicity)
		procaine amide
		quinidine
		lignocaine
		propranolol
		Terminate surgery

Type	Causes	Treatment
Bradycardia	Irritant anaesthetic vapours Drugs: neostigmine suxamethonium digitalis vasopressors C_3H_6, $ChCl_3$ and halothane Overdistension of the lungs in controlled respiration Surgical stimulation of the vagus Traction on extrinsic muscles of eye	Remove offending stimulus IV atropine
AV Block	Cardiac surgery e.g. mitral valvotomy Repair of VSD	Remove offending stimulus e.g. suture involving the bundle of His finger or valvulotome in the heart clamp occluding a coronary artery Insert external or internal pacemaker if AV block is complete and will not respond to drugs such as atropine and isoprenaline
Ventricular Fibrillation	Anoxia Infarction Hypothermia	Adequate oxygenation and CO_2 elimination Cardiac massage Restore myocardial tone with adrenaline or 10% $CaCl_2$ and give 8.4% sodium bicarbonate and 50% glucose Raise temperature, if low Electrically defibrillate. If this fails try biochemical defibrillation (Beveridge & Rollason 1963)

REFERENCES

AGARWAL B.L. & GUPTA C.B. (1967) New X wave in electrocardiographic complex. *Brit. med. J.* **2,** 217

ALLAN C.M., CULLEN W.G. & GILLIES D.M.M. (1961) Ventricular fibrillation in a burned boy. *Canadian M.A.J.* **85,** 432

ALTSCHULE M.D. & SULZBACH W.M. (1947) Tolerance of the human heart to acidosis: reversible changes in RS-T interval, during severe acidosis caused by administration of carbon dioxide. *Amer. Heart J.* **33,** 458

ASHTON J.P. (1965) Dynamic electrocardiography. *World Medical Electronics and Instrumentation,* **3,** 101

AVERILL K.H. & LAMB L.E. (1959) Less commonly recognised actions of atropine on cardiac rhythm. *Amer. J. med. Sci.* **237,** 304

BADERMAN H. & ROBERTSON N.R.C. (1965) Thumping the precordium. *Lancet* **ii,** 1293

BARAKA A. (1968) Safe Reversal (1). Atropine followed by Neostigmine. An electrocardiographic study. *Brit. J. Anaesth.* **40,** 27.

BAY G. & SIVERTSSEN E. (1967) Intracardiac pacing as an emergency treatment in Adams-Stokes Syndrome. *Brit. med. J.* **2,** 199

BAYLEY R.H. (1943) On certain applications of modern electrocardiographic theory to the interpretation of electrocardiograms which indicate myocardial disease. *Amer. Heart J.* **26,** 769

BETHUNE R.W.M. (1965) Precordial electrocardiograph stethoscope. *Anesthesiology,* **26,** 228

BEVERIDGE M.E. & ROLLASON W.N. (1963) Biochemical defibrillation. *Lancet,* **ii,** 1281

BLACK G.W., LINDE H.W., DRIPPS R.D. & PRICE H.L. (1959) Circulatory changes accompanying respiratory acidosis during halothane anaesthesia in man. *Brit. J. Anaesth.* **31,** 238

BOYAN C.P. & HOWLAND W.S. (1961) Blood temperature: A critical factor in massive transfusion. *Anesthesiology,* **22,** 559

BRADLOW B.A. (1964) *How to produce a readable electrocardiogram.* Charles C. Thomas Springfield, Illinois.

BRINDLE G.F., GILBERT R.G.B. & MILLER R.A. (1957) Use of fluothane in anaesthesia for neurosurgery; Preliminary report. *Canad. Anaesth. Soc. J.* **4,** 265

BROMAGE P.R. (1967) Extradural analgesia for pain relief. *Brit. J. Anaesth.* **39,** 721

BUCKLEY J.J. & JACKSON J.A. (1961) Post-operative cardiac arrhythmias. *Anesthesiology,* **22,** 723

136

BURCH G.E. & DE PASQUALE N.P. (1964) *A history of electrocardiography.* Year Book Medical Publishers p. 27

BURNAP T.K., GALLA S.J. & VANDAM L.D. (1958) Anesthetic, circulatory and respiratory effects of fluothane. *Anesthesiology,* **19,** 307

BUSH G.H. (1964) The use of muscle relaxants in burnt children. *Anaesthesia,* **19,** 231

BUSHMAN J.A. (1967) Monitoring the E.C.G. waveform. *Biomed. Engineering,* **2,** 106

CAMPBELL D. (1966) The management of chest injuries. *Brit. J. Anaesth.* **38,** 298

CANNARD T.H., DRIPPS R.D., HELWIG J.Jr. & ZINSSER H.F. (1960) The electrocardiogram during anesthesia and surgery. *Anesthesiology,* **21,** 194

CHOU T.C. & HELM R.A. (1967) *Clinical Vectorcardiography.* Grune and Stratton, London.

CLEMENT A.J. (1962) Atropine premedication for electric convulsion therapy. *Brit. med. J.* **i,** 228

CLIFFE P. (1967) Potentialities of computers in anaesthesia and medicine. *Proc. Roy. Soc. Med.* **60,** 754

CURRIE T.T., CASS N.M. & HICKS J.D. (1962) The scope of surface cooling. An experimental study using quinidine as a prophylactic against ventricular fibrillation. *Anaesthesia,* **17,** 46

DAVIES C.K. (1965) Adrenaline and halothane. *Anaesthesia,* **20,** 374

DAVIES J.N.P. & EVANS W. (1960) The significance of deep S waves in leads II and III. *Brit. Heart J.* **22,** 55

DAWSON B., THEYE R.A. & KIRKLIN J.W. (1960) Halothane in open cardiac operations; a technique for use with extra corporeal circulation. *Anesth. and Analg.* **39,** 59

DELANEY E.J. (1958) Cardiac irregularities during induction with halothane. *Brit. J. Anaesth.* **30,** 188

DOBKIN A.B. (1949) The effects of anticholinergic drugs on the cardiac vagus: I. clinical observations in patients undergoing electro-shock treatment. *Canad. Anaesth. Soc. J.* **6,** 51

DOWDY E.G. & FABIAN L.W. (1963) Ventricular arrhythmias induced by succinylcholine in digitalised patients. *Anesth. and Analg.* **41,** 501

DRISCOLL A.C., HOBIKA J.H., ETSTEN E. & PROGER S. (1960) Myocardial infarction and other E.C.G. changes in the post-operative period. *Bull. Tufts-New Engl. med. Center,* **6,** 1

DUNCALF D., FOLDES F.F., JACOBSON E. & VARGAS P.G. (1965) Investigation of the cardiovascular effects of hexafluorenium. *Brit. J. Anaesth.* **37,** 591

EBNER H., BARCOHANA J. & BARTOSHUK A.K. (1960) Influence of post-spinal hypotension on the fetal electrocardiogram. *Amer. J. Obstet. Gynec.* **80,** 569

EEROLA R., PÖNTINEN P.J. & MIETTINEN P. (1963) Electrocardiographic changes during neurolept-analgesia. *Acta. Anaesth. Scandinav.* **7,** 187

EINTHOVEN W. (1903) Die galvanometrische Registrierung des menschlichen Elektrokardiograms, Zugleich eine Beurteilung der Anwendung des Capillarelektrometers in der Physiologie. *Pflügers Arch. ges. Physiol.* **99,** 472

FARMAN J.V. & JUETT D.A. (1967) Impedance spirometry in clinical monitoring. *Brit. med. J.* **2,** 27

FLUCK D.C. & BURGESS P.A. (1966) A press-stud electrode for continuous monitoring of the electrocardiogram. *Lancet,* **i,** 1405

FOOTE A.V. (1967) Personal Communication

FORBES A.M. (1966) Halothane, adrenaline and cardiac arrest. *Anaesthesia.* **21,** 22

FRASER J.G., RAMACHANDRAN P.R. & DAVIS H.S. (1967) Anesthesia and recent myocardial infarction. *J.A.M.A.* **199,** 318

FRAZER A.K. & GALLOON S. (1966) Intracardiac catheterization. *Lancet,* **ii,** 1133

FRIEDBERG C.J. (1966) *Diseases of the heart,* Vol. 1, 3rd Edit., p. 65. W.B. Saunders, Philadelphia

FUKUSHIMA K., FUJITA T. FUGIWARA T., OOSHIMA H. & SATO T. (1968) Effect of propranalol on the ventricular arrhythmas induced by hypercardia during halothane anaesthesia in man. *Brit. J. Anaesth.* **40,** 53.

GAUTHIER J., BOSOMWORTH P., PAGE D., MOORE F. & HAMELBERG W. (1962) Effect of endotracheal intubation on E.C.G. patterns during halothane anesthesia. *Anesth. and Analg.* **41,** 466

GILSTON A., FORDHAM R. & RESHNIKOFF L. (1965) Anaesthesia for direct current shock for the treatment of cardiac arrhythmias. *Brit. J. Anaesth.* **37,** 533

GLOVER W.E. & SHANKS R.G. (1967) Massive overdosage of adrenaline. *Brit. med. J.* **ii,** 293

GOTTLIEB J.D. & SWEET R.B. (1963) The antagonism of curare: the cardiac effects of atropine and neostigmine. *Canad. Anaesth. Soc. J.* **10,** 114

GRANT I.M.V. (1966) Treatment of status asthmaticus. *Lancet,* **i,** 363

GROGONO A.W. (1963) Anaesthesia for atrial defibrillation. Effect of quinidine on muscular relaxation. *Lancet,* **ii,** 1039

HART D.D. & DUTHIE A.M. (1964) The effect of chloroform and halothane administration on the liver. *Proc. III Congr. Mund. Anaesthesiol.* **2,** 86

HEARD J.D. & STRAUSS A.E. (1918) A report on the electrocardiographic study of two cases of nodal rhythm exhibiting R-P intervals. *Amer. J. med. Sci.* **155,** 238

HERON J.R. & ANDERSON E.G. (1965) Concomitant cerebral and cardiac ischaemia. *Lancet,* **ii,** 405

HEWITT P.B., HOOD P.W. & THORNTON H.L. (1967) Propranolol in hypotensive anaesthesia. *Anaesthesia,* **22,** 82.

HILL D.W. (1966) The use of radiotelemetry in the monitoring of babies. *Acta Anaesth. Scand. Proc. III, Second European Congr. Anaesthesiol.* p. 127.

HILL I.G.W. (1932a) Cardiac irregularities during chloroform anaesthesia. *Lancet*, **i**, 1139

HILL I.G.W. (1932b) The human heart in anaesthesia; an electrocardiographic study. *Edinb. med. J.* **39**, 533

HON H. (1965) Fetal electrocardiography. *Anesthesiology*, **26**, 477

HUDON F. (1961) Methoxyflurane. *Canad. Anaesth. Soc. J.* **8**, 544

HUGHES C.L., LEACH J.K., ALLEN R.E. & LAMBSON G.O. (1966) Cardiac arrhythmias during oral surgery with local anesthesia. *J. Amer. Dent. Ass.* **73**, 1095

HUTCHINSON B.R. (1967) Electrocardiographic changes in children following extubation. *Med. J. Austr.* **1**, 151

INKSTER J.S. (1966) A monitoring probe for use in paediatric anaesthesia. *Anaesthesia*, **21**, 111

JACKSON P.W. & WOODHEAD Z.M. (1967). Propanidid anaesthesia for electroconvulsive therapy. *Anaesthesia*, **22**, 704.

JACOBSON E. & ADELMAN M.H. (1954) The electrocardiographic effects of intravenous administration of neostigmine and atropine during cyclopropane anesthesia. *Anesthesiology*, **15**, 407

JENKINS A.V. (1966) Electrocardiographic findings during bronchoscopy. *Anaesthesia*, **21**, 449

JOHNSTONE M. (1950) Cyclopropane anaesthesia and ventricular arrhythmias. *Brit. Heart J.* **12**, 239

JOHNSTONE M. (1951a) The heart during vinyl ether anaesthesia. *Anaesthesia*, **6**, 40

JOHNSTONE M. (1951b) Pethidine and general anaesthesia. *Brit. med. J.* **ii**, 943

JOHNSTONE M. (1953) Adrenaline and noradrenaline during anaesthesia. *Anaesthesia*, **8**, 32

JOHNSTONE M. (1956) Electrocardiography during anaesthesia. *Brit. J. Anaesth.* **28**, 579

JOHNSTONE M. (1966) Propranolol (Inderal) during halothane anaesthesia. *Brit. J. Anaesth.* **38**, 516

JOHNSTONE M. & NISBET H.I.A. (1961) Ventricular arrhythmia during halothane anaesthesia. *Brit. J. Anaesth.* **33**, 9

JONES H.D. (1968) Heart block in hyperbaric oxygen, *Lancet*, **i**, 822.

JONES R.E., DEUTSCH S. & TURNDORF H. (1961) Effects of atropine on cardiac rhythm in conscious and anesthetised man. *Anesthesiology*, **22**, 67

KATZ L.N. & PICK A. (1956) *Clinical electrocardiography. Part I.* Lea & Febiger, Philadelphia, p. 507

KATZ R.L. (1964) Antiarrhythmic and cardiovascular effects of synthetic oxytocin. *Anesthesiology*, **25**, 653

KATZ R.L. (1965) Epinephrine and PLV-2. Cardiac rhythm and local vasoconstrictor effects. *Anesthesiology*, **26**, 619

KATZ R.L., MATTEO R.S. & PAPPER E.M. (1962) The injection of epinephrine during general anesthesia with halogenated hydrocarbons and cyclopropane in man 2, Halothane. *Anesthesiology*, **23**, 597

KAUFMAN J.M. & LUBERA R. (1967) Pre-operative use of atropine and electrocardiographic changes. *J.A.M.A.* **200**, 197

KAUFMAN L. (1966) Cardiac arrhythmias during dental surgery. *Proc. Roy. Soc. Med.* **59**, 731

KAVAN E.M. & KOLVIN R.C. (1965) Clinical use of an esophageal E.C.G. electrode during surgery—modification of the esophageal stethoscope. *Anesth. and Analg.* **44**, 20

KENDALL B., FARRELL D.M. & KANE H.A. (1962) Fetal radioelectrocardiography: a new method of fetal electrocardiography. *Amer. J. Obstet. Gynec.* **83**, 1629

KENNEDY B.R., DUTHIE A.M., PARBROOK G.D. & CARR T.L. (1965) Intravenous regional analgesia: An appraisal. *Brit. med. J.* **i**, 194

KERR J.H. (1967). Intravenous regional analgesia (A clinical comparison of lignocaine and prilocaine). *Anaesthesia*, **22**, 562.

KERWIN A.J., MCLEAN R. & TAGELAAR H. (1960) A method for the accurate placement of chest electrodes in the taking of serial electrocardiographic tracings. *Canad. med. Ass. J.* **82**, 258

KING B.D., HARRIS L.C.Jr., GREIFENSTEIN F.E., ELDER J.D.Jr. & DRIPPS R.D. (1951) Reflex circulatory responses to direct laryngoscopy and tracheal intubation performed during general anesthesia. *Anesthesiology*, **12**, 556

KÖLLIKER A. & MÜLLER H. (1856) Nachweis der negativen Schwankung des Muskelstroms am natürlich sich contrahirenden Muskel. *Verh. phys.-med. Ges. Würzb.* **6**, 528

KRISTOFFERSEN M.B. & CLAUSEN J.P. (1967). Bradycardia and hypotension during cyclopropane anaesthesia caused by hyoscine as premedication. *Brit. J. Anaesth.* **39**, 578.

KRONSCHWITZ VON H. (1964) Direkt auf die Brustwand aufzusetzendes Kardioskop. *Anaesthesist*, **13**, 170

KRUMBHAAR E.B. (1918) Electrocardiographic observations in toxic goiter. *Amer. J. med. Sci.* **155**, 175

KURTZ C.M., BENNETT J.H. & SHAPIRO H.H. (1936) Electrocardiographic studies during surgical anesthesia. *J. Amer. med. Ass.* **106**, 434

DE LANGE J.J. (1963) Cardiac arrest with halothane and adrenaline. *Anaesthesia*, **18**, 537

LARKS S.D. (1961) *Fetal electrocardiography*. 1st edn. Charles C. Thomas, Springfield, Illinois

LARSON A.G. (1964) Deliberate hypotension. *Anesthesiology*, **25**, 682

LAZAR M.R. & SNIDER E.A. (1966) New hemostatic agent for geriatric gynecology. *Obstet. gynec.* **27**, 341

LEPESCHKIN E., MARCHET H., SCHROEDER G., WAGNER R., DE PAULA E., SILVA E. & ROAB W. (1960) Effect of epinephrine and norepinephrine on the electrocardiogram of 100 normal subjects. *Am. J. Cardiol.* **47,** 594

LEVY A.G. (1914) The genesis of ventricular extrasystoles, under chloroform with special reference to consecutive ventricular fibrillation. *Heart,* **5,** 299

LEWES D. (1965) Multipoint electrocardiography without skin preparation. *Lancet,* **ii,** 17

LUPPRIAN K.G. & CHURCHILL-DAVIDSON H.C. (1960) Effect of suxamethonium on cardiac rhythm. *Brit. med. J.* **ii,** 1774

LURIE A.A., JONES R.E., LINDE H.W., PRICE M.L., DRIPPS R.D. & PRICE H.L. (1958) Cyclopropane anesthesia; cardiac rate and rhythm during steady levels of cyclopropane anesthesia in man at normal and elevated end-expiratory CO_2 tensions. *Anesthesiology,* **19,** 457

MABLE S.E.R. (1966) Electrocardiograms by telephone. *Biomedical Engineering,* **1,** 262

MALSTRÖM G., NORDENSTRÖM B., NORLANDER O. & SENNING A. (1960) The coronary patient as an anaesthetic risk. Results of anaesthetic procedures for coronary angiography with a technique including periods of hypotension. *Acta anaesth. scand. Suppl. VI,* p. 24

MARTIN K.H. (1958) Die Wirkung des Succinylcholins auf den Herzrhythmus. *Atti XI Congr. Soc. ital. Anest.* p. 362

MATTEO R.S., KATZ R.L. & PAPPER E.M. (1962) The injection of epinephrine during general anesthesia with halogenated hydrocarbons and cyclopropane in man. 1. Trichlorethylene. *Anesthesiology,* **23,** 360

MATTEO R.S., KATZ R.L. & PAPPER E.M. (1963) The injection of epinephrine during general anesthesia with halogenated hydrocarbons and cyclopropane in man. 3. Cyclopropane. *Anesthesiology,* **24,** 327

MAZZIA V.D.B., ELLIS C.H., SIEGEL H. & HESHEY S.G. (1966) The electrocardiograph as a monitor of cardiac function in the operating room. *J.A.M.A.* **198,** 103

MCARDLE L. (1959) Electrocardiographic studies during the inhalation of 30% CO_2 in man. *Brit. J. Anaesth.* **31,** 142

MCLISH A. (1966) Diazepa as an intravenous induction agent for general anaesthesia. *Canad. Anaesth. Soc. J.* **13,** 562

MILLEDGE J.F. (1965) A new axis-deviation calculator. *Lancet,* **ii,** 954

NICHOLSON M.J. (1966) Potential danger of intravenous concentrated potassium penicillin G. Case history. *Anesth. and Analg.* **45,** 474

NOBLE M.J. & DERRICK W.S. (1959) Changes in the electrocardiogram during induction of anaesthesia and endotracheal intubation. *Canad. Anaes. Soc. J.* **6,** 267

NOORDIJK J.A., OEY F.T.I. & TEBRA W. (1961) Myocardial electrodes and the danger of ventricular fibrillation. *Lancet,* **i,** 975

ORR, D. & JONES I. (1968). Anaesthesia for laryngoscopy. A comparison of the cardiovascular effects of cocaine and lignocaine. *Anaesthesia,* **23,** 194.

ORTH O.S. (1958) In *Pharmacology in Medicine*. 2nd edn. Chapters 5 & 6. Ed. V.A.Drill. McGraw-Hill, New York

ORTON R.H. & MORRIS K.N. (1959) Deliberate circulatory arrest: The use of halothane and heparin for direct vision intracardiac surgery. *Thorax*, **14**, 39

OSBORN J.J. (1953) Experimental hypothermia; respiratory and blood pH changes in relation to cardiac function. *Amer. J. Physiol.* **175**, 389

PANDIT S.K. & PANDIT R. (1965) Occulo-cardiac reflex under general anaesthesia and the use of gallamine as a preventive measure. *Ind. J. Anaesth.* **13**, 80

PARKER J.B.R. (1965) Some observations on the foetal heart during labour. *Proc. Roy. Soc. Med.* **58**, 634

PAYNE J.P. & PLANTEVIN O.M. (1962) Action du fluothane sur le coeur. *Anesth. and Analg.* **19**, 45

PHIBBS B. (1966) Central venous pressure monitoring—localisation of a catheter with teflon wire. *New Eng. J. Med.* **274**, 270

PITTS F.N., DESMAROIS G.M., STEWART W. & SCHABERG K. (1965) Induction of anesthesia with methohexital and thiopental in electroconvulsive therapy and clinical observations in 500 consecutive treatments with each agent. *New Eng. J. Med.* **273**, 353

PÖNTINEN P.J. (1966) The importance of the oculo-cardiac reflex during ocular surgery. *Acta Ophthal.* (København) Suppl. 86

POOLER H.E. (1957) Atropine, neostigmine and sudden deaths. *Anaesthesia*, **12**, 198

PRICE H.L., LURIE A.A., JONES R.E., PRICE M.L. & LINDE H.W. (1958) Cyclopropane anesthesia: epinephrine and norepinephrine in initiation of ventricular arryhthmias by carbon dioxide inhalation. *Anesthesiology*, **19**, 619

PRINZMETAL M., CORDAY E., BRILL I.S., SELLARS A.L., OBLATH R.W., FLIEG W.A. & KRUGH H.E. (1950) Mechanics of the auricular arrhythmias. *Circulation*, **1**, 241

RIDING J.E. & ROBINSON J.S. (1961) The safety of neostigmine. *Anaesthesia*, **16**, 346

RICHARDS C.C. & FREEMAN A. (1964) Intra-atrial catheter placement under electrocardiographic guidance. *Anesthesiology*, **25**, 388

ROBINSON J.S. (1964) Profound hypotension for radical surgery in malignant disease of the face. *Symposium on induced hypotension in surgery*. Cambridge, 21st November

ROLLASON W.N. (1957) Atropine, neostigmine and sudden deaths. *Anaesthesia*, **12**, 364

ROLLASON W.N. (1958) Side effects of antidote drugs. *Atti XI Congr. Soc. ital. Anes.* p. 546

ROLLASON W.N. (1964) Halothane and phaeochromocytoma. *Brit. J. Anaesth.* **36**, 251

ROLLASON W. N. (1965) The monitoring of hypotensive anaesthesia. *Anaesthesia*, **20**, 479

ROLLASON W.N. (1967a) Intravenous anaesthesia in dentistry, *Dental News*, **4**, 1.

● ROLLASON W.N. (1967b) The role of the anaesthetist in the treatment of cardiac arrhythmia. *Proc. I Anaesthesia*, '66, p. 495.

ROLLASON W.N. (1968) Diazepam as an intravenous induction agent for general anaesthesia. *Diazepam in Anaesthesia* (Ed by P.F.Knight & C.G.Burgess). John Wright, Bristol, p. 70.

ROLLASON W. N. & DUNDAS C. R. (1966) Recent developments in out-patient dental anaesthesia. *Acta. Anaesth. Scand. Proc. II, Second European Congr. Anaesthesiol.* p. 207

ROLLASON W.N. & DUNDAS C.R. (1968) E.C.G. changes during dental anaesthesia (In Press).

ROLLASON W.N., DUNDAS C.R. & MILNE R.G. (1964) E.C.G. & E.E.G. changes during hypotensive anaesthesia for 'no catheter' prostatectomy. *Proc. III Congr. Mund. Anaesthesiol.* **1**, 106

ROLLASON W.N. & HOUGH J.M. (1957a) Electrocardiographic studies during endotracheal intubation and inflation of the cuff. *Brit. J. Anaesth.* **29**, 363

ROLLASON W.N. & HOUGH J.M. (1957b) A possible fallacy in single lead electrocardiography. *Lancet*, **ii**, 245

ROLLASON W.N. & HOUGH J.M. (1958) Thiopentone induction and the electrocardiogram. *Brit. J. Anaesth.* **30**, 50

ROLLASON W.N. & HOUGH J.M. (1959) Some electrocardiographic studies during hypotensive anaesthesia. *Brit. J. Anaesth.* **31**, 66

ROLLASON W.N. & HOUGH J.M. (1960a) A study of hypotensive anaesthesia in the elderly. *Brit. J. Anaesth.* **32**, 276

ROLLASON W.N. & HOUGH J.M. (1960b) Is it safe to employ hypotensive anaesthesia in the elderly? *Brit. J. Anaesth.* **32**, 286

ROLLASON W.N. & LATHAM J.W. (1963) Anaesthesia for intracranial aneurysms. *Anaesthesia*, **18**, 498

ROLLASON W.N. & PARKES J. (1957) Anaesthesia, hyperventilation and the peripheral blood. *Anaesthesia*, **12**, 61

ROSE G.A. (1961) A calliper for siting the precordial leads in electrocardiography. *Lancet*, **i**, 31

ROSEN M. & ROE R.B. (1963) Adrenaline infiltration during halothane anaesthesia. *Brit. J. Anaesth.* **35**, 51

ROSS E.J. PRITCHARD B.N.C., KAUFMAN L., ROBERTSON A.I.G. & HARRIS B.J. (1967) Pre-operative and operative management of patients with phaeochromocytoma. *Brit. med. J.* **1**, 191

RUMBALL C.A. (1963) An axis-deviation calculator. *Lancet*, **ii**, 20

SAGARMINAGA J. & WYNANDS J.E. (1963) Atropine and the electrical activity of the heart during induction of anaesthesia in children. *Canad. Anaes. Soc. J.* **10**, 328

144 ELECTROCARDIOGRAPHY

SCHAMROTH L. (1966) *An Introduction to electrocardiography*, pp. 12, 41, 83. Blackwell Scientific Publications, Oxford

SCHAMROTH L. & CHESLER E. (1963) Phasic aberrant ventricular conduction. *Brit. Heart J.* **25**, 219

SCOTT J.C. & BALOURDAS T.A. (1959) An analysis of coronary flow and related factors following vagotomy atropine and sympathectomy. *Circul. Res.* **7**, 162

SEUFFERT G.W. & URBACH K.F. (1967) Influence of thiopental induction on incidence and types of cardiac arrhythmias during cyclopropane anesthesia. *Anesth. and Analg.* **46**, 267

SHENKER L. (1966) Fetal electrocardiography. *Obstet. & Gynec. Survey*, **21**, 367

SMYTH C.N. (1962) Foetal response to adrenaline and noradrenaline. *Brit. med. J.* **i**, 940

SMYTHE P.M. (1963) Studies on neonatal tetanus and in pulmonary compliance of the totally relaxed infant. *Brit. med. J.* **i**, 565

SOLWAY J. & SADOVE M.S. (1965) 4-Hydroxybutyrate—a clinical study. *Anesth. and Analg.* **44**, 532

STEWART J.S.S., STEWART W.K., MORGAN H.G. & MCGOWAN S.W. (1965) A clinical and experimental study of the electrocardiographic changes in extreme acidosis and cardiac arrest. *Brit. Heart J.* **27**, 490

STRUNIN L. (1966) Some aspects of anaesthesia for renal homo-transplantation. *Brit. J. Anaesth.* **38**, 812

SUTTIN G.J. & HEESE H.deV. (1964) Electrocardiogram in idiopathic distress syndrome of newborn. *Lancet*, **ii**, 532

THOMAS E.T. (1965) The effect of atropine on the pulse. *Anaesthesia*, **20**, 340

TOLMIE J.D., JOYCE T.H. & MITCHELL G.D. (1967) Succinylcholine danger in the burned patient. *Anesthesiology*, **28**, 467

USUBIAGA J.E., GUSTAFSON W., MOYA F. & GOLDSTEIN B. (1967) The effect of intravenous lignocaine on cardiac arrhythmia during electroconvulsive therapy. *Brit. J. Anaesth.* **39**, 867

WALLER A.D. (1887) A demonstration on man of electromotive changes accompanying the heart's beat. *J. Physiol.* **8**, 229

WALTS L.F. & PRESCOTT F.S. (1965) The effects of gallamine on cardiac rhythm during general anesthesia. *Anesth. and Analg.* **44**, 265

WATERS R.M. (1951) *Chloroform: a study after 100 years*. Madison, Wisconsin

WAY W.L & LARSON C.P. (1967) Recurarization with quinidine. *J. Amer. Med. Ass.* **200**, 153

WEISS W.A. (1960) Intravenous use of lidocaine for ventricular arrhythmias. *Anesth. and Analg.* **39**, 369

WHITBY J.D. (1963) Electrocardiography during posterior fossa operations. *Brit. J. Anaesth.* **35**, 624

WYNANDS J.E. & BURFOOT M.F. (1965) A clinical study of propanidid (F B A 1420). *Can. Anaesth. Soc. J.* **12**, 587

INDEX